WOMEN AN

HEALTHCARE FOR WOMEN SERIES

WOMEN AND SEX

Anne Hooper

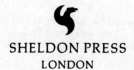

SHELDON PRESS
LONDON

First published in Great Britain in 1986 by
Sheldon Press, SPCK, Marylebone Road, London NW1 4DU

Second impression 1988

British Library Cataloguing in Publication Data

Hooper, Anne
   Women and sex.—(Healthcare for women)
   1. Women—Sexual behaviour
   I. Title   II. Series
   306.7′088042   HQ29

   ISBN 0-85969-516-6
   ISBN 0-85969-517-4 Pbk

Photoset by WBC Print Ltd, Bristol
Printed in Great Britain by
Whitstable Litho Ltd, Whitstable, Kent

Contents

Introduction: Starting Points

This book is written for women who know something has gone wrong with their sexual response and fear that this is affecting the quality of their emotional life. It covers all age groups, from the teenager who may have had a bad first experience of sex and is therefore afraid of making further sexual relationships, to mature and older women, both married and unmarried.

As sexuality is often seen as an expression of emotional health, it can be hard to know where to begin tackling the problem when a sexual relationship starts breaking down. Is it the poor sex, in a physical sense, which is responsible? Or is it the feelings behind the sex?

To help women sort out this dilemma for themselves, this book covers all aspects of sexual problems. By understanding what happens to us physically, we are then better able to look at the emotional side of sex. As a result of doing this, we may realise that it is our emotions and not just physical problems, that are getting in the way of sexual happiness. But it can work either way.

When I lost interest in sex, at the age of twenty-one, I was extremely worried. I didn't welcome my doctor's general preamble about 'phases of life', I wanted information on what might be going on inside me and how it began. At the age of twenty-two I worked out for myself that the pill (in those days in extremely high dosage) was probably responsible for my lack of response. The solution was then easy. I adopted an alternative method of contraception. Since then, there has been much fascinating research compiled on health aspects of sexuality, a great deal of which I refer to. There is still need, however, for a lot more.

If I could have looked up 'lack of desire' in those days and skimmed down a list of physical and emotional possible causes, I would have been a happier and more knowledgeable woman, sooner. But at that time such a book did not exist. Neither did

1

suggestions about what to do about your problem once you had firmly understood it. Surprisingly, although there is a plethora of sex manuals, such a volume still doesn't exist for women outside the medical profession. There are many general sex books with beautiful drawings but not one that explores every known cause of sexual difficulty in women and provides specific medical advice and detailed self-help programmes. This book aims to provide that much needed information in an easy-to-understand and accessible way.

When I was struck down with what used to be called 'frigidity', *all* sex problems were thought to be in the mind. Fortunately, thinking has changed since then. We are now aware that some difficulties are due to physical changes within the body. We are aware, too, that the body and the mind interact so closely that they are virtually indivisible. So, do we concentrate on the hormones first and hope that if we sort these out sexual feeling will be regained? Or do we learn to relax, relying on the theory that relaxation aids our sexual drive?

Some women become so confused by the various possibilities that they cannot find a way into the problem at all. However, years of experience with women's sexuality groups have taught me that it doesn't matter *where* you start. The important thing is to begin. *Any* way into a problem is a help. It's a bit like doing embroidery: as long as you eventually cover the entire area with stitches, it does not matter in the slightest where you started. This book begins with the most basic problems in our sex lives—including topics such as lack of orgasm and lack of desire. I cover all the possible causes: marital conflict, hormonal disorders, physical illness, lack of confidence, drug reactions, etc. and explain the most up-to-date methods of help, including self-help.

The second part of the book concentrates on problems of sexual health, and examines the effect that the various types of contraception may have upon your life, how ill-health may affect sexual desire, how some drugs, even commonplace ones, can alter sexual response. During the years of maturation, women experience many bodily changes. Puberty, menstruation, pregnancy, lactation, birth, menopause can all affect our feelings about making love. How these do so is also examined in this section.

2

Introduction

I did not want to include a specific chapter on lesbianism in a book entitled 'sexual problems' for I don't see lesbianism as a problem but as a state of being. However, like anyone else, lesbians have sexual problems. Although, in the main, these problems are much the same as those of any other woman, there are a few situations which are more often experienced by lesbian women—hence Chapter 10.

The number of violent sex crimes increases frighteningly every year and ways of dealing with the emotional after-effects are suggested here. So, too, are ways of coping with grief and with the onset of old age and how this affects our sexual images of ourselves.

Finally, although many self-help methods are listed in these pages, sometimes sexual deadlock demands more than self-help. With this in mind, the appendices list both self-help programmes and helping agencies.

By clearly listing the causes, effects, research and up-to-date helping methods of treatment, I hope readers will understand the choices open to them. *Women and Sex* is intended to provide a clear pathway but allow you to choose in which direction to travel. By receiving specific information about a particular problem, we give ourselves insights into our sexuality from which we can hopefully move on to improve the quality of our whole life.

PART 1

Problems of Sexual Response

ONE

Lack of Orgasm

Orgasm is the delightful culmination of sexual arousal. All the mental and physiological enjoyment which goes into love-making comes to a climax—a spilling over of sensual feeling. Physiologically, orgasm consists of a series of vaginal contractions which are a reflex reaction to the build-up of sexual tension. Subjectively, climax is a peak of intense physical pleasure.

Orgasm is experienced during intercourse, during masturbation and occasionally during dreams or fantasies. It most commonly needs privacy and peace in which to take place but has surprised some women by unexpectedly occurring on top of the bus, in the launderette or even in the office. Some women have to be in a distinctly languorous mood to have a climax; others find that they can be tired, cross, or even angry, and it still happens. However, this chapter is concerned with those of you for whom it does not happen or for whom it only happens in special circumstances.

Some women who complain that they do not experience orgasm, actually mean that while they are easily orgasmic during self-masturbation, they cannot have an orgasm during intercourse with their partner. Because they believe that orgasm is only of value when experienced in the 'proper way' (i.e., during intercourse) they discount their very real but private experience.

The problem is not so much a sexual one as a social one. First they need to understand their climactic experience *is* valid. Secondly they want, though they do not necessarily need, to be able to transfer their ability to climax from masturbation to love-making.

The greatest obstacle to this is the necessity to ask a partner for specific sexual behaviour. Such are the repressions placed upon us from girlhood that the simple act of request can be excruciatingly hard to carry out. The partner, the circumstances and our self-esteem need to be very favourable indeed for some of us to be able to do this. We can, however, learn.

7

Women who never experience orgasm

By far the largest group of women with sex difficulties is that of women who have *never* experienced orgasm. And this group divides into three different types of orgasmic problem:
- Organic problems such as hormonal disturbance, impaired physiological response, disease and drug reaction.
- Psychological difficulties which affect the ability to climax although not always the ability to experience arousal.
- Generally unresponsive for reasons not yet clearly understood (about 8 per cent).

Let us examine these problems more closely.

Organic causes

Hormonal disturbances can affect our sexual response in a variety of ways:
- Lack of certain hormones can directly subdue response to touch, or can affect the amount of oestrogen in the body. This latter, in turn, may reduce vaginal lubrication so that genital stimulation is painful rather than pleasurable and thus impedes orgasm.
- Some biochemists theorize that inadequate amounts of androgen in the female body prevent both the physical growth of the genitals and the development of erotic sensation. (Androgen is the hormone that produces male sex characteristics in men, and also affects female sexual development.)
- A heightened prolactin (milk-producing hormone) level can subdue sexual response, as can sometimes the pill.
- Some biochemists believe that an over-high level of progesterone (the hormone that causes changes in the secretions of the uterus during menstruation and pregnancy) can influence mood by creating depression which among many other things, greatly reduces sexual libido. (For further details please turn to Chapter 6 on Hormones and Sex.)

Impaired physiological response. Not much is understood yet about organic reasons for poor sex, but an interesting recent realization is that some women with impaired sexual response may be suffering from a similar condition to that of men with erectile problems. Because women are easily able to have intercourse without visible signs of arousal, this condition has been previously obscured.

While the reasons for arousal problems are often psychological (as discussed in this chapter and in Chapter 2) a small minority of men with arousal problems suffer from a physiological blockage or leakage. Something impedes the blood flow to the penis and therefore prevents erection, or causes the blood to seep out of the penis as soon as it gets there. If there are analogous situations for women it may be that some women (and it must be emphasized only a very few would fall into this category) might benefit from very sensitive surgery. As yet these are speculations for the future; no doctor specializing in sex problems has turned this theory into fact.

But I keep remembering a study of 103 men in Nanterre, France, who were investigated by means of ultrasound. Seventy-six of them were found to have organic reasons for their inability to erect. In particular the majority suffered from a leakage of blood supply to the penis. Sixty per cent of these men underwent surgery and regained their potency.

Diseases such as multiple sclerosis, temporal lobe epilepsy, and chronic kidney failure may be directly responsible for impairing or subduing sexual response. Illnesses which result in general poor health, depression, constant pain or fear of exercise may indirectly affect sexual responses. (For more details see Chapter 9.)

Drug reactions which affect either ability to climax or to be generally sexually responsive are listed in Chapter 8 on drugs and sexuality. Sometimes the drugs are medically prescribed for illness which, otherwise, would lead to a dangerous deterioration in overall health. But drug addicts such as those on heroin and methadone also find their sex lives are affected.

All these physiological causes need expert diagnosis in order to determine what may be responsible for them. Sometimes problem drugs can be withdrawn and alternatives prescribed which do *not* affect sexual response. In the case of depression, however, drug treatment may be necessary to help overcome the depression before the sufferer is able to respond to sex therapy. Before you undertake sex therapy you would be wise to find out whether or not organic causes lie at the root of the trouble since, if there are organic causes, no amount of well-meaning counselling will help.

Psychological problems

Ignorance. This is hardly a psychological problem but it amounts to such when we have no idea what is causing our difficulties. Even today, many men and women don't understand very basic facts about sex. Discussion and reading can help overcome this. (See Appendix 2 on p. 173, for suggested reading list.)

Lack of self-esteem. Sexual confidence is closely bound up with feelings about oneself. If, for any reason, we feel inadequate, this low self-esteem affects our attitude towards sex. We feel hopeless about it before we begin and when these feelings are communicated to a partner, he rapidly learns not to expect too much of us.

It may be that we dislike our body and how it looks. Perhaps the contemporary ideals of how women should appear have made us acutely self-conscious about our body shape and we shrink from exposing it. Some women fear that their genitals are deformed through sheer unfamiliarity with what a mature woman's genitals look like.

A lack of self-esteem may affect how we deal with life. Some women are naturally assertive, almost unconsciously having picked up from those around them a firm mode of behaviour that gets results. Others have not had the same intuitive skills or opportunities.

The practice of simple assertion skills allows us to become effective with those around us and as we begin to achieve what we aim for this creates an upward spiral of confidence which extends to other aspects of life, including sex. It gets easier, for example, to persevere at learning to masturbate in order to experience orgasm for the very first time. It becomes possible to talk about sex with a partner when previously you had never dared. Introducing masturbation into intercourse through new assertive self-confidence leads to orgasms during intercourse for the first time. Learning assertion is one of the most important sex aids women can use.

Members of the Women's Sexuality Workshop use the YES/NO assertion exercise. In it they have to say YES to three things they really want to do and NO to three things they really don't want to do (in one week). The exercise can be interpreted on a very simple level, such as whether or not to eat a chocolate bar or, on a much deeper level, such as whether or not to ask your live-in lover to leave. It is an exercise capable of changing your life, however uncertain you may be feeling right now.

Parental example—'teaching'. The kind of relationship our parents have with each other affects our own expectations of love and sex. If your parents gave ample demonstrations of their affection by cuddles and hugs, then the odds are you will have learned a warm and tactile way to behave with your partner. If, on the other hand, they were not close, or constantly insulted each other and actually warned you off having sex 'because of the awful consequences', theirs is an exceedingly bad model from which to build your own loving partnership. If you do not know how to demonstrate affection you are handicapped. Learning to hug, learning to say 'I love you' once a day as a deliberate exercise, can sometimes save a marriage. Learning to enjoy physical closeness without this necessarily leading to intercourse paradoxically improves lovemaking when it does take place.

The feminist view of sexism. As girl children and adolescents we are traditionally taught to provide pleasure for others—in particular, men. We learn to be supportive wives, house-keepers, mothers, secretaries, etc. But we don't learn that we, too, deserve to have time and attention spent on giving us pleasure. Boys are not taught to pay this special caring to us nor are we taught to devote time to self-pleasuring. Yet before we can love men wholeheartedly we need to love ourselves wholeheartedly.

This is specially relevant to sexual response. We tend to expect that men will provide us with our sexual responses because we have been taught this way. We often traditionally assume that he will make all the first moves, will know what to do in bed and will generally sweep us off our feet, teaching us everything we need to know.

The reality is often different. After all, it is unreasonable to expect a man to know what turns us on if we don't know that ourselves. Women do not all have identical sexual responses. Each one of us is highly individual and what works with one woman will not necessarily work for the next.

Learning to know our own sexual responses therefore removes the responsibility from where it has been rather unfairly placed, on men, and puts it firmly on to us. Once our responses are familiar to us, we are in a far better position to communicate them to a partner during lovemaking.

Learning to masturbate through a self-pleasuring programme is one route to achieving this. Introducing newly-learned masturbation into lovemaking can result in orgasms being experienced together for the first time. Learning to climax in this way can lead on to climaxes being experienced during intercourse, with or without masturbation.

Fear of being overwhelmed. One of the most common complaints from women who have not yet climaxed is something they describe as 'automatic cut-off'. They enjoy lovemaking, become aroused, feel themselves nearing a peak and then, just as they are almost at orgasm, something cuts off and the sensations go.

Automatic cut-off nearly always happens as a result of anxiety. The most common reason for this is a fear of being overwhelmed in some way. Some fear that they will lose consciousness, actually faint. Others are terrified of losing control, or of what they may look like during such extreme sensations. Rehearsing imagined loss of control can sometimes help overcome these anxieties. Understanding exactly what does happen during orgasm can also be an aid. (Very few women *do* faint, although it has been known.) What generally happens is that, although the brain transports you to a different level of consciousness during orgasm, it is possible to descend from that level any time you choose. If you suddenly needed to be in control (perhaps because the baby cries) you would instantly return to reality, ready to leap to its defence. You do not actually lose consciousness—you just change it.

Some women overcome automatic cut-off by thinking of something else, focusing on sexy thoughts or an erotic fantasy. Some view sexy pictures or literature in order to transcend the cut-off. Others find that a more intense stimulation sometimes sends them into an orgasm. Use of a vibrator can be helpful. A vibrator is an electrically operated sex aid which provides strong stimulation.

Women who experience this cut-off problem only in the presence of a partner but who are fine during masturbation, need to practise nearing orgasm with him in a series of stages. If you can masturbate to orgasm in his presence that is a good start. He can hold you and cuddle you while you are doing so and gradually become incorporated as part of your masturbation routine so that eventually both of you are able to have intercourse while he simultaneously masturbates you.

If even this is impossible because of the inhibition you feel in his presence, then the following exercise might be helpful:
1   Moving into the next room, you might try masturbating there, with the door shut between you.
2   On the next occasion you might do the same but this time with the door open.
3   On a third occasion, you might masturbate near the doorway (still open), then in the doorway, then in his room and so on until eventually you have got used to masturbating in his presence and are able to do so lying next to him on the bed. From there both of you can continue with the former procedure.

If you find it easier to respond to your partner's touch rather than your own, then learning to incorporate *his* methods of masturbating *you* may also overcome automatic switch-off.

Sex is 'dirty'. If our upbringing has taught us that sex is 'dirty', this can make us ashamed of our natural sexual inclinations. We may even shrink from sex. Discussing these attitudes with other women and broadening our knowledge about sex will help us to relax. Exploring sexuality with a partner, very slowly and with constant reassurance, taking lovemaking in a series of stages, can also help us to be more comfortable. A return to old-fashioned courtship is almost prescribed!

Sex is illicit. If sex is forbidden it acquires an illicit thrill for some and occasionally becomes such an established part of a sex pattern that the only really good sex is that which contains an element of risk. As a result, some women are only ever able to experience orgasm with a lover (and not with a husband). Some couples overcome the problem by turning it into a game, making special appointments to have sex with each other in places other than their home. Other couples accept that sex with a legal partner may never be as thrilling as that with a lover but learn to respond nevertheless, using the above methods of extra stimulation.

Dislike of body secretions and smells. Sometimes the 'sex is dirty' attitude, includes an aversion to natural body odours and secretions. Both men and women can be helped to overcome these feelings with a mild behaviour therapy in which each is encouraged to feel comfortable about the other's genitals. Self-help includes looking at each other's genitals in detail, each displaying their genitals as they might a non-sexual part of their body. Doing this with the aid of a mirror, touching and smelling each other's secretions, learning every part of the genitals and what their role is, is all part of the familiarization process.

Women can be encouraged to look closely at ejaculate while both sexes would gain useful information by keeping a menstruation diary for her. Changes in vaginal secretion should be noted in it, as well as mood changes during the menstrual month.

Misbeliefs. Sexual behaviour abounds with myths:
- If you masturbate too much you'll grow tired and ill before your time.
- Masturbation weakens your body.
- Women who want sex often are unnatural.

Examining beliefs about sexuality with others is a useful exercise. Sometimes the myths strike at our very identity: 'The only true orgasm is one experienced during sexual intercourse', is particularly destructive since some women who so far have only experienced orgasm through masturbation, genuinely believe they are inadequate human beings. Yet this is nonsense.

Faking orgasm. Many women who fake orgasm do so because they believe that if their partner knew the awful truth (i.e., that they don't climax) their partner will leave them. Rather than risk this, they suffer sensual deprivation instead. If you never reveal to a partner that his lovemaking doesn't work for you, you never give him the chance to alter the sexual pattern to suit you better. You trap yourself with your fear. Not unnaturally, he continues with the pattern you have condoned because he believes it to be successful.

The only way out of this dilemma is for you to learn about your sexual response through self-pleasuring and then to explain it to your partner with suggestions for re-structuring your lovemaking. This is a very sensitive negotiation and rehearsing all eventualities can go a long way to making it an easier experience.

Lack of privacy. The fear of interruption is a destructive one and if it is a very real one (i.e., you are living in crowded conditions) it is not always easy to overcome. This fear does not, however, hold everyone back. This indicates that lack of sexual response in such situations is an inhibition as much as a real fear.

The Women's Sexuality Workshop habitually gives instruction in how to fit a simple bolt to the bedroom door. This expedient is glaringly obvious yet strangely enough often hesitated over. 'Strange' because the very act of locking the door induces a sense of security and privacy and may be what tips the scales to sensual enjoyment.

Much of the hesitation comes from the anxiety that family or friends or relations will want to know why you are being private. While it may not *always* be appropriate to give a straight answer, this is often a very satisfactory way of getting the peace that you want. An excellent illustration of this comes from a story told by a friend who, when on holiday in France with his family, packed the children off to the beach and retired into the family caravan with his wife to make love.

Unfortunately, his ten-year-old daughter decided to return. After several times unsuccessfully shouting through the door that she should go away, her father finally yelled in desperation 'Mummy and I are making love. Go away please.' Whereupon his daughter said 'I'm sorry Daddy. I'll come back in half an hour shall I?' and went away. She was quite capable of understanding her parents' need for privacy when it was spelled out. Desperate lovers please take note!

Fear of pregnancy. This fear can cause such anxiety that it clouds all lovemaking and prevents any response. The simple answer is to obtain satisfactory contraceptive advice. Family Planning Clinics and Brook Advisory Centres will help you to choose suitable and reliable contraception, and there are very few people who cannot use some form of birth control. Now that these options are open reasonably easily to both men and women, if such an option is regularly *not* taken up, this may be a very strong message indeed about your sexual feelings:

- It may indicate that you fear being a sexual person and sub-consciously choose to obstruct your sexual response.
- It may indicate that although you think you ought to be having a sexual relationship, at a deeper level you don't really want it.

Since the unwitting victim of such confusion is an unwanted child, women recognizing this dilemma would be wise to seek personal counselling.

Partnership problems. There can be so many of these it is impossible to list them all. Here are just a few:

- Partner's ineffective lovemaking technique. Women commonly say that *they* have a sex problem which is ruining their *husband*'s sex life. Investigation shows, however, that the problem may be shared or occasionally caused entirely by the husband. A classic example is where the 'frigid' wife is sent in by the husband to be 'fixed' by the sex therapist. Learning self-pleasuring does indeed 'fix' the wife—she becomes orgasmic and realizes at the same time that she might have done so years ago if her husband had been the great lover he claimed to be. When she returns to her husband 'fixed', his reaction is to retreat into impotence. She has been carrying both her own *and* his sex problem. Solving her problem has revealed his. He is the one who now needs help.
- Partner's lack of caring. Poor sex can be the consequence of a partner's lack of thought and care for your needs. You can't force someone to care for you. You might be able to help them change by getting them to examine their attitude and what it is doing to the relationship, but there is a limit to how much *one* partner may do to improve a relationship. If the other person consistently refuses to work with you, it may be less stressful in the long term to face up to the fact that the relationship is emotionally dead.
- Partner's male chauvinism. Quick intercourse without fore-play may not necessarily indicate that your sex partner is an unfeeling narcissist, nor that he lacks caring. He may be

poorly educated in the ways of loving or conditioned to certain beliefs. How much his chauvinist attitude can be altered will depend largely on how deeply the attitude constitutes part of his sense of identity as a man. Many men may be very responsive to requests for a different sexual style. They simply need to be asked. If, however, your partner's attitudes about men and women's places in the world are rigid and inflexible, the prospects are not rosy.

• Pressure from partner to climax. If a man's enjoyment of the sex act is lessened by an inability to bring his woman to climax, he may feel inadequate. His feelings of failure then place a burden of guilt upon his partner. Even as she tries harder for his sake to climax, the guilt increases her inability to relax and enjoy herself. One method of self-help is to stop trying to reach orgasm and, instead, just enjoy the sensuality of lovemaking. (See Appendix 1 on p. 167.)

• Anger over money/children/etc. Sex therapy will help very little until the anger has been expressed, listened to and solutions found. If this can be managed, sex usually spontaneously improves. Anger which builds up over the years into deep-seated resentment is far harder to resolve, but the process is similar.

• Lack of interest in sex. A natural difference in libido is one of the hardest sex problems to resolve. The urge for sex isn't something to be forced and, although couples lacking in desire may be able to work on rekindling their sexual feeling (see Chapter 2), if it was never really there in the first place, there is little hope for alteration. Other options may need to be seriously considered, such as:

1 Lovemaking sessions which don't include intercourse
2 Relying on masturbation
3 Finding other sexual partners.

A superbly loving husband may be able to make all the non-sexual aspects of marriage so rewarding that enduring the pangs of frustration is worthwhile until such a time as your own sexual desire fades. Any marriage where sexual expression is denied outlet will have to be quite remarkable in other ways in order to survive. But some can and do.

External stress. Stress at work can become focused on marital problems, resulting in lack of sex or poor sex. When such

confusion arises, work and home stresses need to be dis-
entangled before the sex problems can be resolved. Some
couples manage this without help. Others only need to have the
overlap of work stress pointed out to improve sexual relations.
There are specialist counselling organisations for men and
women with career stresses which get out of control. (See
Appendix 2 on p. 173.)

Unequal 'growth'. Personal development cannot be neatly regulated to match that of our partner. Sometimes one partner may
acquire a new perspective on the world and seeks to change his
or her lifestyle in a way that is unacceptable to the other—who
is still content with doing things the old way. The situation can
create so much anger that sex becomes impossible. A classic
case is the shy woman who becomes confident as the result of
ten years as an efficient wife and mother—very different from
the hesitant and timid person she used to be. Meanwhile, her
husband, who started married life as teacher, provider and
father figure *hasn't changed.*

If such a marriage is to continue she needs to give her
husband time in which to catch up while he must realize he has
got to change. If both these compromises are made then the
relationship stands a good chance of improving maritally and
sexually. This kind of change can be made through constant
discussion, assurances of love and a commitment to the
relationship. It is likely to be painful but, ironically, it is the
feelings of pain which compel both partners to compromise.
The compromise must be *wanted* (as opposed to grudgingly
given) so that angry feelings are allowed to dissipate and love
and sex may be expressed again.

Feelings of personal insecurity. Some of us are so wounded by
childhood experience or early love affairs that we feel under
constant permanent 'threat'. Husband or boyfriend may represent our only security, with the result that we cling to them in a
stifling manner. We are nevertheless unable to experience
climax because of a deep distrust. Rebuilding the foundations of
personal security when they have been undermined is a slow
process. The best way is through a solid and committed
partnership with someone who understands your emotional
needs, and can withstand clinging behaviour while continuing

to be loving. As real trust in such a partner develops, so too can sexual trust. Women who have not been orgasmic previously may then feel self-confident enough to become so.

Not every man is such a saint of course, but talking through past insecurities may give a partner in this situation insight into your clinging behaviour and consequently lend him patience and tolerance. Mutual masturbation and self-pleasuring exercises can help too, provided any difficult or unpleasant emotions these may reveal are paid attention. If these can be regarded as part of a 'working through' process and reassurance given, they—as well as the exercises themselves—can create trust and the desired response. If couples need help with the process, personal counselling can assist. (See Appendix 2 on p. 173.)

Performance pressures. Some of us find during intercourse that we are so acutely aware of what we are doing that we are watching ourselves. This vision (of ourselves) impedes our internal concentration on erotic sensation so that we become blocked in our sexual response. Learning to focus on the sensual experience through mutual 'pleasuring' exercises, and to substitute sexual fantasy for 'spectatoring' can help us across this hurdle.

Fear of pain. Whether this fear is based on real or imagined pain the effect is much the same:
- If the fear is imagined, then the painful fantasy needs to be explored (with husband, lover or therapist) so that we are helped to come to terms with what the 'worst' might be. (See *Fear of being overwhelmed*, page 12, for further details.)
- If the pain is real because of a physical condition, the poor sexual response usually spontaneously recovers when the condition has been treated or naturally improves. Certain positions help sexual response for sufferers from such conditions as arthritis etc. (See Chapter 4 on Painful Sex.)

Orgasm occasionally or rarely experienced

Strangely, women who have *occasionally* experienced orgasm often have greater difficulty in learning to do so *regularly* than do women who have never experienced it at all. One explanation might be that the greater the body's ability to climax, the greater might be the mind's resistance. In other words, women who know they are capable of climax but can't manage it often may possess deeper layers of anxiety about their sexual identity than others. The more they realize they *are* sexy, the more they subconsciously apply sexual control.

Some women require a specific 'aid' to subdue their anxiety long enough to let their erotic feelings have full reign. Alcohol or drugs which work directly on removing inhibition can improve some women's sex lives. But alcohol or drugs are not a satisfactory long-term answer since too much alcohol or a drug can impair response rather than promote it. More natural methods of achieving relaxation are preferable.

Possible causes

Most of the psychological causes and some of the organic ones applicable to women who have *never* experienced orgasm (discussed in the first half of this chapter) are also relevant to women who occasionally experience orgasm. Some causes, however, may prove more intense or deep-seated. The following causes are additionally implicated:

Anxiety and tension. Some of us, from earliest childhood, are tense for no easily identifiable reason. Our tension may reflect a neurogical irregularity or may be the result of early trauma. As we mature, this tension overlaps into other areas of life including sexuality. Attempts to overcome the tension (by self-help or with a partner) may serve to increase the tension through lack of success—and a vicious spiral sets in.

Some women may so fear failure or being ridiculed that they cannot relax at all. Others may paradoxically fear success, in that they fear, if they allow themselves to be sexual, they will in some way be threatened.

Finding out what these 'internal' threats are is the key to self-help. It is only by 'removing' threats that we are encouraged to relax and enjoy ourselves. An important point is that even if someone is habitually anxious or tense, not everyone with these problems reacts sexually by repressing orgasm. There seems to be an extra ingredient here of learned inhibition.

Some women find that bio-energetic bodywork (exercises to enable energy to flow through the limbs) helps them relax their bodies, and liberates sexual energy for the first time. Bio-energetic exercise coupled with deliberate recall of past emotional events help some women to work through their tension and find sexual enjoyment.

For example, Heather's bio-energetics brought her Presbyterian grandfather's disapproval strongly to mind. Sexual movement made her feel in some way incestuously dominated by him. Exercising in a class, however, helped her to discover her normal sexy feelings and accept herself as a sexual person. After this she experienced orgasms although she still found it hard to relax.

Distrust of a specific partner. Some women are able to respond happily to sexual stimuli with one partner and not with another. The reasons for this may be chemical (your partner has the wrong smell!) or intuitive in that you are able to sense there is something not quite right even if you are uncertain what that is. If he happens to be your first sex partner it is very easy to imagine that you are sexually handicapped—forever. A subsequent partner, however, may show you this was your reaction to a specific person rather than a regular reaction to sex.

Religious conditioning. Some religious sects indoctrinate their members with a particularly repressive and punishing view of sex. If, as a young and impressionable teenager, you were or are threatened with hell-fire should you 'rashly' attempt to follow what feel like normal impulses, you may find yourself caught in a destructive struggle between your conditioning and natural desire. Work in women's groups has shown that the best way to overcome such divisive feeling is with encouragement and strong support from other women and/or friends. Experiencing orgasm and discovering the sky *doesn't* fall on your head is a wonderful experience! Use of a vibrator can also be very helpful here.

A need for more stimulus. Some women may have experienced orgasm in the past without understanding how. A self-pleasuring programme which includes using a vibrator may help them to understand the process of sexual excitement and orgasm better, and provide them with much more stimulus than previously experienced. A vibrator can be of help both in teaching women to discover their response and to transfer this response into a relationship.

Some women feel strongly that orgasm is not complete unless it is accompanied by the closeness of a partner's body and a feeling of being filled by his penis. If however, orgasm doesn't always happen this way, masturbation in addition to the sex act can provide the extra stimulation needed without detracting from the feeling of being filled.

Orgasm with no sensation

A few of us experience orgasm with no feeling: we don't know we have climaxed because there has been no sensation. Work with a vibrator and mirror can help us to *see* that we *are* climaxing. If you are a woman like this, sometimes there is such relief at actually seeing climax (even without sensation) that you will be encouraged to carry out the self-pleasuring exercises in Appendix 1 on p. 167. But these need to be combined with careful thought about why your mind may be putting such a block on sexual expression with a partner. The current explanation of the condition is that it is caused by intense anxiety which can anaesthetize sexual response. If it is indeed a case of mind over matter, counselling may be of assistance. However, there are also possibilities that the condition may be caused by organic damage or a hormone irregularity. (See Chapters 6, 8 and 9.)

Orgasm as pain

Another form of unsatisfactory orgasm is when pain builds up and orgasm is consequently unpleasant. This can be altered by individual experimentation with masturbation. Self-stimulation, either by hand or, more easily, with a vibrator covered with a layer of silky material to lessen the stimulation, is often surprisingly helpful. Some women find direct stimulation of the clitoris is too intense and need something far more gentle and gradual.

Fear of strong stimulation, based on previous bad experiences, may also be responsible for converting sensations into pain rather than pleasure. Relaxing and taking things easy with a self-pleasuring routine (see Appendix 1) can usually overcome your pain.

Other ways to orgasm

Here are some of the other ways in which some couples achieve orgasm, all of which may take some getting used to, or you may reject as not for you.

Oral sex

How can you get used to it if you don't like it but your partner does? Gentle encouragement to practise and to spend a little longer on each practice session may eventually result in pleasing oral sex for you and your partner. But if, having tried, you dislike the activity, then don't do it. No one should be forced to do anything sexual they find distasteful. Exactly the same, of course, applies to him if you happen to like cunnilingus and he does not.

Anal intercourse

This is another activity that arouses strong reactions. First, it is strictly illegal between heterosexuals although not between consenting homosexuals. This reflects an anomaly in our sex laws rather than active practice of the law. It is some fifty years since the last anal sex prosecutions relating to heterosexuals were heard.

Again, the main sex problem which arises from this practice is active dislike. If you hate anal sex then you certainly should not participate. If, however, you are willing to experiment but find it difficult, gentle manual stimulation and a lot of lubrication should prepare the body for penile penetration. If it hurts, the reason is undoubtedly because you are tense. If you are able to relax, penetration will be much easier. If this does not happen you should listen to what your body is telling you—it really does not want this kind of sexual activity.

Masturbating your partner

Just as many women enjoy being masturbated by their partner, so too do many men. But what if you don't like masturbating your partner? Often women feel like this because they are inexperienced and fear being inadequate at giving their man pleasure. Asking what pleases him, allowing yourself to be guided are the best ways of learning. Ask him to give you time and positive feedback. There are no general rules for this very personal activity between two people. Once again, however, if after giving it a fair try, you dislike the practice, it is wise to find something else that works better for both of you.

Experimenting with different lovemaking positions

Many women starting on their sex life feel deeply inhibited about this. In most circumstances, just getting to know and trust a partner allows us to relax and be a little more daring. But if this doesn't happen and inhibition becomes a problem it helps to look back into family life and see where such guarded attitudes may have come from. Often a strongly religious background can cause sexual repressions which block lovemaking.

Self-help consists of deliberately familiarizing a partner with your body and with touch. This needs to be done slowly and sensitively, with massive reassurance for you and a great deal of patience on his part. It needs to be carried out at *your* pace. The self-pleasuring exercises in Appendix 1 on p. 167, both for you alone and for the two of you together, are excellent ways of slowly introducing trust and sensuality.

Should you find the most sensitive of sexual exercise impossible, however, it is important to go back over former repressive experiences and fears and talk them through. If this is difficult to do, between the two of you, do enlist help from a sex therapist. Joining a women's sexuality group, too, can be an excellent way of coming to terms with uneasy feelings about sex. (Lists of sex therapists and women's groups are given in Appendix 2 on p. 173.)

Multiple orgasm

Most women wouldn't reckon this to be a problem. But some women worry deeply about being inadequate if they *can't* manage more than one orgasm. It is important to come to terms

with the fact that we are all very different sexually. What
be easy for one, isn't for the next. It has nothing to do wit
being inadequate. We simply possess different strengths of
sexuality according to our upbringing, our hormones and how
we happen to be feeling at the time. A few people find that they
can have multiple orgasms with a vibrator but not in any other
way. Whether you can or cannot doesn't matter.

Variety of orgasmic experience

It is natural to think that the first orgasm you ever experience
sets the pattern for all orgasms to come. And if it is not a very
satisfactory one it can be disturbing enough to make further
orgasms even less satisfactory. Yet one woman's orgasmic
experience over the years can be extremely varied. She may
experience some deeply satisfying orgasms and at other times
find she is unable to climax at all. On one occasion the sensation
may be dilute and fleeting, on another extremely powerful. All
these varied responses serve to show therefore how complicated
is the reason for success or failure.

The knowledge that we *can* climax is a powerful one. It allows
us confidence in our sexuality and an identity as sexual people.
It should enable us to feel good enough about muted climaxes to
allow us, one day, to experience the 'firework display'. If your
first experiences have been disappointing, take heart.

TWO

Lack of Desire

Sexual desire is both a state of mind and (some believe) a chemical response to a desired object. Purists say it is an abstract concept while those who are more down-to-earth associate it with distinct stirrings in places too private to mention! There is at present a debate between sex therapists who say that desire is a separate component of the sexual response pattern and biochemists who state that desire is a matter of hormones.

Whether or not desire can be neatly labelled and put into a category shouldn't matter. But it does. In the past six years, more and more people have arrived at sex therapy clinics complaining that, as a result of their *lack of desire*, their sex life has deteriorated. Such are their numbers that clinical sex therapists have been forced to review the overall pattern of sexual response. Rightly or wrongly, desire is now seen as an important part of the whole process of feeling and being 'sexy'.

One of the most influential 'gurus' of sexual therapy is the therapist Dr Helen Singer Kaplan of New York whose book *The New Sex Therapy* is regarded as a bible by most students of sex counselling. In a further book, *Disorders of Sexual Desire*, Dr Kaplan has offered some new conclusions about women who are unable to muster any interest in sex.

Inhibited sexual desire

Dr Kaplan divides clients lacking in desire (her term for this is 'inhibited sexual desire') into two categories:
- Category one is the woman who behaves as if her sexual circuits are shut down. This woman loses interest in sex, will not make any effort to pursue a sex life and, should an interested and willing partner turn up, will not grasp the opportunity. Possible causes of Category One are thought to be a lack of the necessary brain activity (i.e. a neurological fault) or very early and profound psychological disturbance.

- Category Two (which is more common) covers women whose lack of desire is selective. Either they feel desire and enjoy sex only with certain people or they never actually want or instigate sex but, when stimulated by a partner, are capable of responding.

According to Kaplan, desire is *not* genital but is controlled by the brain. On this basis she has re-defined the sexual response cycle that human sexual response does not consist of four phases as previously defined by Masters and Johnson flowing spontaneously one to another but rather that it is made up of three individual and distinct phases. These she calls:

- 'desire', which is a completely new category
- 'arousal' which corresponds to Masters' and Johnson's excitement' and 'plateau' phases
- 'orgasm', which speaks for itself.

The sexual response cycle re-defined

The reason this re-definition is important lies in Kaplan's observation that these three phases can function *separately and apart from each other*. This distinction was *not* perceived by Masters and Johnson and the new description clarifies certain women's orgasmic problems which previously baffled everyone.

To understand Kaplan's idea fully, it helps to see the three sexual response phases in terms of electrical circuitry. 'Orgasm', 'arousal' and 'desire' may be seen as having a common 'generator' in the brain—but each has its own 'circuitry'. And because each phase is separately 'wired', each can go wrong without necessarily affecting the other two. This means a number of sexual combinations are available to women trying to have sex.

- Many women are capable of experiencing desire, arousal and orgasm in one sequence.
- Some women are unable to feel desire but, if stimulated, nevertheless become sexually aroused and experience orgasm.
- Others cannot feel desire or the physical sensations of arousal but are still capable of experiencing the contractions of orgasm. Sometimes these contractions may contain little sensation (as if the genital area is anaesthetized—see Chapter 1); sometimes the orgasm may be experienced as discomfort or even pain, but they are, notwithstanding, still orgasms.

Causes of inhibited sexual desire

The inability to feel desire, says Kaplan, occurs in both men and women and is shown by low libido in both genders. The cause of this is anxiety.

Desire phase problems occur when anxiety is aroused very early in the sequence of desire-excitement-orgasm. In these women the first stirrings of sexual pleasure will evoke anxiety and its immediate defence system—which is to rapidly repress all the feelings of pleasure so far experienced and shut them down. With some of us the anxiety is so deep that 'shut down' can happen at the very thought or expectation of sexual opportunity.

A lack of desire often shows itself as a low sex urge. Those of us who do not feel sexy don't want to make love often. Dr Kaplan notes that patients with desire problems, as a group, tend to have more serious marital/relationship problems than those from other groups, presumably as a result of their lack of interest in sex.

Therapy

Therapy for overall lack of desire

Category One sufferers have a variety of options open to them but a pessimistic outlook. Psychoanalysis may be of assistance; hormone therapy (see Chapter 6) may re-balance the hormone 'mixture' which biochemists believe affects libido. But, so far, results of psycho-therapy have had little effect. There doesn't seem to be much in the self-help line.

Therapy for lack of desire with a specific partner

Much of Dr Kaplan's work has been done with couples who, after a period of marriage, no longer feel desire for each other. As a result their sex life ebbs and each partner becomes disillusioned and bored. Dr Kaplan's therapy programmes attempt to reverse this process and bring sexual feeling back into 'dead' marriages. Not surprisingly, this is very difficult. Only about 20 per cent become orgasmic again.

Getting to the root of anxiety can be hard. The brain may have good reasons for turning off feelings of desire and attempts to turn it on again sometimes amount to re-opening a power station after it has automatically shut down in case of explosion. Burrowing out the root cause therefore needs to be done in a safe atmosphere. It *is* possible for partners to work on this between themselves and below is a list of possible causes which might be explored. (If however the causes are so deep-seated that they don't easily surface, professional therapy may be more useful.)

- Former traumatic sexual experience as a child or teenager, such as rape, indecent assault, or an incestuous experience.
- Fear of becoming so intimate with a partner their mental closeness is a threat that the 'self' will be swamped. Although craving closeness, which is what prompted them to seek the relationship in the first place, an inner part of their ego withdraws from the intimacy of sexuality for 'safety's sake'.
- The state of marriage sometimes confers special anxieties which did not previously exist. For example, some women unconsciously see a husband as a father and therefore lose their desire. Sometimes this change happens after the birth of a baby; when the husband actually becomes a father, the two roles can be confused.
- One partner 'outgrows' the other one over a period of years. The acquisition of new confidence can unbalance the emotional foundations on which the relationship was first built.
- Constant sexual rejection cools sexual feelings.
- Boredom: the sameness of the sex act with the same person, year after year.
- A past hurt perceived by only one member of the partnership. For example, the husband has an affair when the wife expects the first baby. Although both think this is forgiven and forgotten, the birth of the second baby brings doubts and fears back into the wife's unconscious and she can no longer feel sexual desire.
- A sense that lovemaking is a duty. Sex has become a pressurized performance.
- A recent shock. Grief which results in depression can wipe out sexual desire—as can depression of any kind.
- Drug reaction. (See Chapter 8).

Self-help

The level of anxiety provoked by past experiences needs to be examined closely since anxiety is at the root of all the above causes.

Sexual Trauma

Traumatic experiences in the past, such as rape, can leave within the subconscious feelings of outrage, anger, depression, grief, and self-disgust which were not fully expressed at the time. Before you can relax about sexuality you need to uncover these feelings, bring them out and relive them again either with a powerfully supportive partner or a therapist. You need to cry, scream or thump out your rage and grief while being assured that your feelings are justified, acceptable and can be contained.

Containment is a key word here. A rape or incest victim is liable to feel so overwhelmed by a sense of shame and injury that she fears her listeners may be overpowered too and, as a result, reject her. One of the reasons that group therapy by other rape victims or counselling by women involved in rape crisis is effective is because the victim assumes that those who already share her experience will not judge or patronize her. They will be able to *contain* her.

Once she feels 'contained', a mild form of behaviour therapy can be used between sexual partners, instigated and controlled by the woman. (For methods see Appendix 1 on p. 167). Strong feelings, however, may still get in the way of such therapy and they need to be talked through as they arise. A strong 'containing' partner may be able to respond sensitively without outside help. Others, less confident, may prefer to carry out such 'therapy' with the support of a self-help contact or therapist. (See Appendix 2).

Problems thrown up by such work are:
- reluctance on the part of the woman to instigate and take control of the sex act
- early feelings of anaesthesia once desire is awakened
- rage expressed in the shape of violence towards the present and innocent male partner.

It is vital that the real root of these behaviours is recognized, talked about as they arise and 'contained'. Rather than actually accept bodily violence, however, substitute a strong pillow as a butt. This is a stage where it is important to ask for outside advice if the partner finds it hard to cope alone.

Threats to the inner self

These threats are fears, planted by past conditioning and poor experiences, which spring up when the sexual side of a relationship develops. Since the 'threats' are mostly experienced on a subconscious level it can be difficult to establish what they are.

A successful case history. Mr and Mrs P enjoyed a good but occasional sex life when unmarried but living together. Six months after the marriage they were puzzled to find neither felt like sex any more. Intercourse had become an effort. At no time had Mrs P experienced orgasm. Yet she didn't rate this as a reason for 'cooling off'. Neither could perceive any obvious cause. Nothing had gone wrong between them. Sessions with a therapist showed that Mrs P feared sensual success. She had absorbed messages put out by a bitter and depressed mother that sexuality was treacherous and that, in order to retain control over life, it was necessary to be wary of it. As long as Mrs P had remained unmarried she had felt safe. Marriage, however, increases sexual intimacy and her 'safety' reaction had been to shut herself off from all sexual response. (As it was, her anxiety, previous to marriage, had been such that she had never reached a climax.) Mrs P did this 'shutting off' by thinking negative thoughts when it came to intercourse. The problems were compounded by Mr P's similar fear of sensual success. *His* mother had told him that men who wanted a lot of sex were unlovable.

Mrs P was encouraged to work on some self-pleasuring exercises and was gratified to learn she still liked herself after experiencing orgasm this way for the first time. As a result of this breakthrough she recognized that she was partly responsible for her husband's resistance to sex since, up till then, she had held such punishing attitudes towards intercourse. Now she encouraged him to relax in a series of self-pleasuring exercises, similar to those she had done by herself, where intercourse was forbidden.

31

In spite of resistance on his part (which both were able to trace back to Mr P's childhood), they were so heartened by their responses that both felt genuine desire to continue. Mrs P learned to experience orgasm in a combination of mutual masturbation and intercourse, and both partners renewed their interest in lovemaking.

Follow-up a year later showed that other marital problems had got in the way of sex from time to time but that, nevertheless, they had re-established a regular sex life, each *wanting* to make love two or three times a month.

When a partner 'resists'. Couples preferring to identify their inner reasons for lack of desire without therapeutic help may be able to do so by embarking on the sensual pleasuring exercises (see Appendix 1 on p. 167). But these must be combined with frank discussion of the fears that such exercises throw out and careful tracing of their origins. It is also important to recognize that 'resistance'—that is, one partner making it difficult for the 'pleasuring' to continue successfully—needs to be regarded not as resistance to improving the relationship but as an expression of extreme discomfort with something which has happened in the past.

Resistance is an indication that you need to work out what you are feeling and why. Sometimes resistance may simply be an indication that the couple have moved on too quickly through the self-pleasuring exercises and would feel more comfortable going back a step. If the problems seem buried too deep or seem too vague to identify some people will find it easier to seek sex therapy. (For a list of sex therapy sources, see Appendix 2 on p. 173.)

If the lack of desire problems closely follow giving birth, it is a good idea to wait several months before assuming that sex therapy is needed. Extreme fatigue, hormone upheaval, breast-feeding, birth trauma (such as episiotomy—the incision made at the end of the second stage of labour, to ease the actual birth) all depress sexual desire and take time from which to recover. It is also advisable to rule out other physiological changes by seeking a thorough medical examination before assuming that sex therapy is necessary.

Personality growth and change

Years of marriage sees personalities change and mature. Often in a relationship one or both partners may find that they later differ widely from the people they started off as. In some cases the differences may be so great that ending the marriage is the best option. There are many cases, however, which have very good reasons for continuing in spite of this difference—reasons such as a family, or simply that once you re-discover each other's characters and interests, the ties between you may prove more rewarding rather than irksome.

In this instance, deliberately attempting to catch up on each other's interests or to jointly develop new mutual interests and projects re-establishes common ground in fields other than sex. This may also help renew the friendship, and subsequently sexual desire. Examination of present mutual interests may illustrate how a couple's paths have diverged. Deliberate attempts to bring them back on to a shared track could prove to be a new basis for an old relationship.

Individual work on self-esteem through assertion, job challenges or even leisure challenges may help to raise your confidence. Higher levels of self-confidence feed back into the relationship enabling you and your partner to either improve it or to withdraw from it.

If improvement encourages you and your partner to re-discover your sexual relationship, the sensual pleasuring exercises (see Appendix 1 on p. 167) are one way of leading in to this. However, sexual motivation, from both of you, needs to be very strong for the outcome to be sexually successful.

Sexual rejection

Discussion and sensual pleasuring exercises can overcome feelings of rejection, provided that:
- the rejected one gets ample opportunity to bring out and display anger
- the partner is able to acknowledge the problems and is prepared to change
- both continue to want a relationship in spite of the original rejections.

Until this journey has been safely navigated, the behavioural exercises (see Appendix 1) are unlikely to succeed. The key to success lies in the partner's change of heart and unless this exists, attempts to improve sexual intercourse will fail.

Sexual boredom

Returning to 'basics' can be a surprisingly successful activity in marriages of many years where both partners care about each other but are uncertain how to change their sexual pattern.

Some people believe that sexual boredom is best helped by an injection of extra-marital sex of an extrovert kind such as swapping and group sex activities. This belief is usually misplaced, however, since these types of sexual activity can be deeply destructive to all except strong and self-confident relationships where the marital sex continues to be successful.

Returning to 'basics' means a return to the early days of courtship where stroking, caressing and cuddling were usual, and sexual intercourse forbidden.

Former sexual hurt

When a partner, in anger, tells you you are terrible in bed, even if you know he may not have meant it, the doubt festers. Such sexual hurt, based on real or imagined cause, can be ultimately responsible for turning off all sexual desire. In order for sex therapy to succeed, the feelings of hurt need to be expressed, shared, understood and the wounded given reassurance. The partner's ability to accept this implies an openness and willingness to understand and care. However, in marriages where bad behaviour is the root of the problem, this willingness to care doesn't always exist.

If the latter is true the issue boils down to that of incompatibility, and the best option is to separate. But discussion of the incident or attitude which was the root of the problem and an ability to understand and accept that this *was* destructive behaviour, coupled with loving reassurance, can slowly improve lovemaking between partners. Gentle lovemaking with the main focus on *her* pleasure and intercourse delayed or prevented, assists the process.

When sex becomes a pressure

It is very easy in a high-powered and stressful lifestyle to view sex as yet another 'performance pressure'. It may well be delightful when it is actually successful, but the desire to 'give the performance' rapidly wanes. Here are some suggested ways of dealing with it:

- Learn to do with less sex (but make the event a very special time)
- Recognize a constant stress pattern and make deliberate attempts to shed it (if only for two days holiday now and again)
- Enforce a radical change in working life so that stress is halved
- Deliberately set aside full evenings in the week (as would be done for social appointments) for supper, early bath and massage, with sex as optional. This helps remove 'performance' anxieties. The good sensation gained from massage can provide enough incentive to eliminate the idea of having to 'perform'.

Depression

Depression has been mentioned already as a consequence of upheaval or shock. But depression can occur for minor reasons too, yet the side-effects remain the same. It is difficult to feel desire and sexual response when you are depressed. If you are severely depressed, drug treatment may be necessary to lift the depression before you can expect the return of sexual desire.

If depression is part of a small but regular phase of the menstrual cycle it is important to keep a constant awareness about your menstrual dates since this in itself helps women feel more in control of their emotions. Or you might seek PMT therapy. (See Chapter 6.)

Recent work with depressed patients complaining of sexual problems has shown that diazepam (Valium) used in large doses inhibits the patients' response to therapy. If this is prescribed, therefore—which it often is, as a means of aiding depression and restoring sexual feeling—request an alternative.

If you are depressed as the result of grief, *time* is needed in

Women and Sex

which to work out the grief and opportunities should be created in which to talk through sad feelings.

Drug reactions

There are a number of medications and socially used drugs which possess the side-effect of altering sexual response. In some cases they remove sexual desire. For more details see Chapter 8 (drugs table on page 118).

Some women find their desire is selective in that while they can't respond to their husband, they can't stop responding to their lover. Common sense tells us that there is no reason why we should feel desire for everybody and anybody. Because we do not feel desire for one partner does not necessarily mean we will not feel it for someone else. Many desire problems are caused by the unfortunate mistake of choosing the wrong partner.

One of the few good reasons for considering 'surrogate' therapy (in which you are teamed with a specialist partner who can guide you in learning how to have more satisfying sex with your natural partner) is to sort out just such confusions. Dr Martin Cole's patients at the Institute of Sex Education and Research in Birmingham are often able to learn once and for all that they are perfectly functional sexual beings—it just happens to be their chosen partner with whom they are unresponsive.

Another sad fact of love appears to be that passion cannot last for ever. After the first years of a partnership lust inevitably fades, to be replaced by tenderness and companionship. Of course, the demise of passion is not a signal for sex to cease. The majority of couples feel enough warmth and affection for each other to demonstrate their caring by regular lovemaking, but the emphasis is changed from highly-charged desire to a rather lower voltage wish to give and get sensual pleasure with a loved one.

Some of us find it hard to make this transition—the disappearance of passion comes as a shock—a personal rejection. Perhaps, unconsciously, we feel thrown back to the days of childhood rejection when a parent's handling of an explosive situation was less than skilful and we emerged from a family

36

drama wounded. The brain's way of coping with that damage is to close off the pain into a separate compartment, supposedly putting it neatly out of the way. But these are the very people who are super-sensitive to rejection (real or perceived) in later life and who therefore over-react to the natural waning of passion.

It is important to emphasize that the waning of desire in a long-term relationship is probably normal and need not be seen in a negative light. As long as a couple are able to keep sight of the fact that caring and love are rewardingly expressed in sexual intercourse, arousal and orgasm will still be as meaningful and erotic as before even if less often. It is when *all* the components of sexual response disappear (i.e., *desire*, arousal and orgasm) that they may truly be said to have a problem.

Organic reasons for lack of desire

Since no researchers have proved that there *are* organic reasons for lack of desire this section is of necessity short. However, there are grounds for thinking that body chemistry *can* affect all the stages of sexual response.

Biochemist Alan Riley firmly believes that the hormone testosterone is primarily responsible for female desire as well as heightened sexual enjoyment. 'Work carried out by Waxenberg and colleagues in 1950' he says 'show this'.

For further details see Chapter 6 on Hormones and Sex. Where sexual desire is totally lacking it would be appropriate to seek medical referral to an endocrinological specialist for hormone tests.

Sex aids

Work done in women's groups indicates that many of us find it possible to heighten our erotic desire by means of sexually stimulating literature, film material and the use of vibrators. In addition, the regular practice of self-pleasuring exercises, with a special focus on the pleasurable feelings created, can be an acceptable method of growing more comfortable with sex and allaying anxieties concerning it. (See Chapter 1.)

THREE

Difficulties with Masturbation

Woody Allen said that masturbation is having sex with someone you love—a statement ironically relevant to women with difficulties of self-stimulation. For most women, the inability to masturbate is associated with self-confidence. If you feel uncertain about yourself, such uncertainty often prevents you from 'taking risks' in your sex-life. It may also mean that you do not consider yourself worthy of receiving pleasure, especially from yourself. You do not love yourself enough to justify such self-attention.

Masturbation is something we nearly all do unconsciously as little children but we learn very rapidly not to do so. 'It's not nice dear', and 'don't touch yourself there dear, it's dirty', are two common parental messages. In addition, because female sex organs are hidden, a girl has less familiarity with her genitals than a boy. She may not sexually experiment during later childhood like her brother, and it is common for women to discover self-stimulation only in their late teens. Some women *never* discover it, always relying on a partner to provide sexual satisfaction. Despite this, several sex surveys show that around eighty-two per cent of women use masturbation as a regular source of pleasure.

Definition of masturbation

This is the act of stimulating the genitals (in particular the clitoris) in order to generate sexual arousal which may or may not culminate in orgasm. Subjectively, it is described as delightful and fulfilling in its own right. It's a healer, an energy giver, an alleviator of tension, a gift of self-pleasure, and it can be an ecstatic experience when it culminates in orgasm.

Since the experience of masturbation is different for every woman it may be all of those things or it may instead be a very low key affair. If you have anxieties or inhibitions about 'letting go' you may experience a rather muted version of masturbation

38

and orgasm. The following are the most common reasons for inhibition:

- Phobia about touching the genitals
- Ignorance
- Lack of interest
- Belief that such an activity is wrong or immoral
- Deep-seated belief that you are unworthy of receiving pleasure
- Belief that this is a lesbian activity or only 'all right' when done by a male partner
- Belief that it is a sign of immaturity
- Unconscious negative messages derived from parents
- Belief that such activity demonstrates a degraded aspect of the personality.

Reasons for overcoming inhibition

Since most of us expect to experience sexual intercourse at some time in our lives, why then is it desirable to know or to learn how to masturbate?

In general, there is no reason why this should be desirable. Millions of women enjoy sexual fulfilment without having learned to masturbate and provided they are happy with this situation there is no reason why (for them) it should be changed. However, there are some weighty arguments in favour of the activity.

- Observations show that many children learn to masturbate spontaneously at an early age—in some cases as early as the first month of life. Thirty-six per cent of one-year-old infants were reported to play with their genitals. Between the ages of two and three, many more masturbate. These are indications that experiencing sexual activity is *natural* to a very large number of all children and that masturbation is a quickly learned activity that enhances the body's natural sexual reflexes. It is only as the children get older that masturbatory behaviour ceases, and it is a fair guess that this is the result of learned inhibition.
- Learning your individual sexual response via masturbation enables you to feel comfortable with it and to gain sexual-self-confidence.

- Such familiarity allows increased likelihood of successful transition to sexual encounters with a lover.
- Sexual self-knowledge allows you to take responsibility for your own orgasm. When a partner lacks the knowledge, when you are partnerless, and as a means of gaining some insight into your partner's response, this is invaluable.
- It is an intensely pleasurable activity.
- It gives a long term sexual relationship the best alternative means by which to survive should intercourse prove difficult or impossible.

How to overcome inhibition

1 Attempt to understand the circumstances which led to masturbation becoming taboo for you. Was there anyone to talk to as a child or teenager about sex—any friend or sibling with whom to compare notes? If not, perhaps you never had the chance to learn. Did your parents' attitude affect your feelings? Often the women who attend sexuality groups have parents who rarely or never showed affection for each other, rarely kissed or hugged and never, never talked about sex to the children except to make it clear that it was undesirable.

Has your sex role been responsible for soliciting double-standard messages about sexuality? As women we are often taught to deny ourselves pleasure. True pleasure is often selfish and as the 'caring' sex it is our role to supply pleasure to others, not to expect it for ourselves. On this basis, are you able to be selfish enough to concentrate on yourself and your feelings of sexuality in the single-minded manner needed to allow you to masturbate to orgasm? Since our sensuality—and especially our orgasm—can be experienced only by us and no one else, it is reasonable that we need to concentrate on our own feelings during sexual activity. Thinking of how glorious this must feel to your partner may be pleasant—but it won't do a lot for your clitoris.

2 Get to know your body and its responses through simple, private erotic exercises (see page 167). In a daily programme which continues for at least six weeks learn to massage yourself, relax in a sweet smelling bath, take time off to spoil yourself by doing anything that really catches your fancy. As the weeks go by, the self-massage includes genital exploration,

re-awakening of genital sensation and learning to build on unfamiliar or half-forgotten sensations of pleasure.

3   Learn to use sex aids such as vibrators and sexual fantasy. Erotic literature can assist women who need to learn to fantasize.

4   Accept a massage from someone else.

5   Read recommended literature on self-pleasuring (see page 173).

6   Learn to be more assertive about life in general. A useful simple assertion exercise used by women in sexuality groups is the YES/NO exercise. (See Chapter 1 for details.)

Masturbation as a sex aid

While it does not really matter that seventy per cent of women cannot climax solely as a result of intercourse, it certainly would matter if they could not experience some form of sexual enjoyment with their partner. This is where masturbation comes in. As well as being a delightful experience in its own right, it can be used as a major part of lovemaking, allowing *both* partners to reach orgasm together.

Biologically, one of the original functions of orgasm was to encourage sexual encounters between men and women for the purpose of reproduction. But female orgasm was not strictly necessary for this. It may have evolved as a safeguard against destructive aggression. It relaxes our bodies when otherwise they might be subject to tension. It thus acts as a biological device for making us easier to live with. Masturbation, as a pathway to orgasm, is a way of using that device.

There are a number of methods with which to combine intercourse and masturbation. One of the most satisfying methods is to stimulate the clitoris either by hand or by vibrator during intercourse. Either one of you can do the stimulating, and the great advantage of this method is that you are able to climax containing your lover.

Other methods include him stimulating you either before or after intercourse or you stimulating yourself while held closely and encouraged by your lover. Some of us find that by learning to climax through combining masturbation with intercourse we eventually learn to climax during intercourse *without* needing masturbation. Others who cannot respond to someone

41

else's stimulation are pleased nevertheless to share a good sexual experience with the partner they love.

Alfred Kinsey (1954) and Shere Hite (1974) discovered from their surveys of women, that while around thirty per cent of women are able to climax during intercourse, eighty-two per cent regularly achieve orgasm through masturbation. Such was the discrepancy between these figures and the popularly held belief that the 'normal' way to climax was during intercourse, that we have been forced to reconsider what women's 'normal' sexual response is. Many people now think it is more 'normal' to be orgasmic through masturbation than it is through intercourse. For many, the combination of the two is the answer to sensual happiness.

Masturbation myths

Contrary to repressive folklore, masturbation does not make you blind, deaf, give you 'flu, send you insane or kill you. Nor does it mean that all women who practise masturbation are nymphomaniacs. This last old wives' tale is interesting, however, in that it may have been, in earlier years, the women with a higher sex drive who dared take masturbation 'risks'. These same women may also have been the most active ones sexually and would therefore have been vulnerable to innuendo and slander.

Mrs Whitehouse and many others influenced by early psychological theory see masturbation only as a stage of sexuality which is normally experienced during childhood and teens. Should you continue to masturbate at a later date, these people believe there is something abnormal about such prolonged practice or that you are stuck at a childhood stage of development. Of course there *are* cases where masturbation is an expression of an abnormal condition but for the vast majority masturbation is a comfortable, independent and normal addition to a range of sexual activity available to us, at any age and any stage.

Some women fear that to practise masturbation indicates that they are confirmed spinsters, the implication being that only women who are unable to get satisfaction from a partner would resort to self-stimulation. If, for any reason, you don't have a partner, masturbation is a very enjoyable and valid method of giving yourself pleasure. *There is nothing wrong in giving yourself pleasure.* Neither is there any law, biological or otherwise, which says we may only receive pleasure through a partnership. Nor does such activity indicate you are not also capable of enjoying other sexual experiences. You cannot overdo masturbation. (Some people fear they will get addicted to it.) But research has shown that the body can only take so much and eventually reaches a stage where it is incapable of continuing; it then forces you to stop.

Others fear that by experiencing orgasm through masturbation they may not be able to do so through intercourse. There is no way of knowing if this is the case since we can never tell 'what might have been'. But some women are able to learn to masturbate in different patterns, to masturbate during intercourse and to alter their sexual activity so that they are able eventually to become orgasmic during intercourse. The desirability of possessing this as a goal, however, needs to be questioned, as explained below.

Patterns of masturbation

There is no set way in which one 'ought' to masturbate. Instead, masturbation patterns depend on the way in which each of us discovers the activity. Our styles of masturbation are uniquely our own. Many women have always masturbated since they were small girls and perhaps developed their pattern by rolling on an object such as a teddy bear. Their adult pattern therefore might consist of rolling, face down, on a pillow or hot water bottle. Some discover masturbation through clenching, then letting go of their thigh muscles. Others come to orgasm by contracting, and then letting go of their perineal muscles (those in the vagina and pelvic floor). It is easy to see that the last three patterns would be difficult for their owners to incorporate with intercourse. If this becomes a goal therefore, it is sometimes necessary to learn other ways of masturbation, and very often use of a vibrator is one method of doing so.

Some women need to move their bodies in order to feel sensuous. Others like to lie as if dead while only their hand works. One woman may find her body flutters all over like a leaf during extreme excitement and that, as an extension of this, her orgasm vibrates every inch of her. Another may find it impossible to respond to genital stimulation but climaxes explosively when her ears are tickled. Everyone needs a period of experimentation (both on their own and with a partner) to find out what is satisfactory and what fails dismally.

Masturbation as a marital problem

However open you may be about masturbation this doesn't, alas, guarantee that a partner will be similarly comfortable. It can be an unpleasant shock for your partner, if inhibited, to discover that you happily engage in self-stimulation. Your activity gets translated into a threat. By giving yourself orgasms, you can be seen to be depriving your partner of sex he considers rightfully his.

If you have been reluctant to have sexual contact, your partner may be perfectly justified in having that reaction. Your masturbation could be a means of avoiding having intercourse. But it could also begin a useful discussion which allows you both to air your feelings and improve the situation.

Solitary masturbation can be used as a method of punishment, as a means of staving off intimacy or as the means to enjoy a fetish. Men, more commonly than women, get attached to forms of sex where the exciting sex object is not a human being but more usually an object. Porn magazines can be used this way, as can ladies' underwear and so on. The possessor of the fetish has to want the relationship to endure very strongly indeed in order to be able to regulate such masturbatory activity.

If, however, self-masturbation is being enjoyed as a happy extra and there is not only no secret about it but your partner is actively invited to join in, then his adverse reaction reflects his own 'hang-ups' about sex and *not* a righteous fear about his relationship with you.

The situation may be more complicated, however. If one partner (say the woman) is very inhibited, has never learned to masturbate and as a result has no knowledge of her own sexual response, those inhibitions can communicate themselves uncomfortably to the partner, whose response may be to masturbate.

Sometimes he may masturbate because the woman has not yet learned to be sexual in her own right and her inhibition turns lovemaking into an ordeal. It isn't much fun making love with someone who is passive to the point of 'doing her duty' and lies on the bed like a log. On the other hand, it takes two to create an atmosphere of trust—and trust is what such a passive partner needs in order to improve.

The easy-sounding solution is that you should learn to masturbate in order to become aware of your sexual response and to then take that new knowledge about excitement and orgasm into shared lovemaking. But if you are deeply inhibited, you have to want to change your attitude very strongly indeed before you are able to make the necessary moves.

Patience, an ability to inspire trust and constant tactile reassurance are some of the qualities your partner needs in this situation. Sensitive information about lovemaking, either from a book or pamphlet may also be helpful, but there is also a danger that the knowledge that many other people have no inhibitions at all may only reinforce the feelings of inadequacy. Long-term, patient loving and a gentle build-up to erotic feeling are the best ways of helping someone enjoy sensuality.

A tiny percentage of women possess a very low libido (drive to obtain sensual satisfaction). As a result, they are *never* very interested in sex. Many of them may be willing (and pleased) to have intercourse but are not capable of obtaining much pleasure from either intercourse or masturbation. (See Chapter 2 on Lack of Desire and Chapter 6 on Hormones and Sex.)

How to masturbate

One of the key mistakes men make in trying to masturbate their partners is to focus entirely on the vagina. It is in fact, the tiny bud-like clitoris which is responsible for most of the good sensations women experience during lovemaking. It acts both as a receiver and a transmitter of sexual feeling.

Some women stimulate the whole of their genital area and not the clitoris alone. Others massage their entire body before reaching down to the pelvis. Some caress a nipple with one hand while concentrating on their clitoris with the other. Others find that the clitoris becomes painful if it is manipulated too hard or for too long. They might react with more pleasure to light fingertip-twirling and circling on the apex of the clitoris. Very few women manipulate the head of the clitoris directly; mainly they stimulate one side of the clitoral shaft. For the female orgasm to continue, once it has begun, stimulation has to go on until the climax is completed.

If the stimulation is too strong, it may be better done through a layer of light material such as a silk scarf or a thin, soft towel. If the clitoris becomes painful after a while, additional lubrication such as saliva, KY jelly or a vegetable-based massage oil usually helps.

If sensation becomes anaesthetized, this might indicate that anxiety has been aroused or that the procedure has become boring. Use of sexual fantasy is one way of overcoming these problems. Exploring reasons why sexual success is an issue also helps.

Women who can't masturbate to orgasm

In theory, all of us are capable of masturbation but not every one of us is capable of masturbating to orgasm. While the majority of women are able to learn this, there remains a small percentage of women (8 per cent) who are not able to do so. For further details see Chapter 1.

Just as there are a few highly sexed individuals, there are also some lowly-sexed ones. It is normal for these latter not to want much sexual activity; this includes masturbation. There is nothing wrong with having a low sex urge; this just happens to be some people's sexual identity. A general lack of interest in sex is not, in itself, a problem. It only becomes one within the context of a marriage where the other partner finds it unacceptable. There is everything right with leading a celibate life as a single person if that is what you feel happy with.

Masturbation as neurosis

Since the practice of masturbation is more accepted today, the concept that it is a neurotic form of behaviour has necessarily had to change. Most forms of masturbation are now regarded as normal.

But there are a few cases where excessive masturbation, combined with other neurotic characteristics, may be abnormal. For instance, a woman who habitually masturbates in

46

the office or on the train, is, by present day standards, abnormal. Usually this kind of public display is accompanied by other disturbed behaviour, and such an individual needs psychiatric treatment.

Where to get help

Women's centres sometimes know of women's sexuality groups specializing in 'non-neurotic' sex therapy. Some hospitals run sexuality groups in their psychological departments (GP referral is usually needed). Some women set up their own groups. Free-lance sex therapists help both single women and couples. (See Appendix 2 on p. 177 for details.)

FOUR

Painful sex

Dyspareunia or painful intercourse is experienced by both sexes but, in particular, by women. Discomfort can have either physical or psychological causes—or both. If there is a likelihood of vaginal infection, uterine disease or inadequate surgery, then medical advice should be sought without delay. The following are all common causes of painful intercourse.

Lack of lubrication

When you are sexually aroused, vaginal lubrication (the flow of natural secretions from the vaginal wall) is a sign that you are ready for intercourse and one of the earliest indications of sexual arousal. If this lubrication is missing, not only will intercourse be very uncomfortable but the entire genital area will be unprepared.

Accompanying vaginal secretion, there should be a slight enlargement of the vulva and lower vaginal tissue due to engorgement with blood. (This is not unlike the swelling experienced by men which leads to erection.) Also, the vaginal entrance should open in readiness for the penis. None of these things happen if arousal is impaired, which means the quality of sexual intercourse is affected. Therefore, the cause of this lack of arousal needs investigation.

A basic ignorance of sexual technique can be the cause. Lack of stimulation due to ignorance can be resolved by seeking information from a sex education book or from a sex counsellor.

Where poor sexual technique is at fault, discomfort is sometimes increased by folds of skin and vaginal hair being pushed into the vagina during penetration. This is specially likely to happen if you have large inner labia or luxuriant pubic and labial hair. The simple solutions are to trim the hair and to separate the labia with fingers (either his or yours) before penetration.

Lack of stimulation through laziness is a rather different problem. The lazy partner needs to acquire an urgent understanding of how his laziness affects the relationship over and above sex. If, after careful and tactful discussion, he still cannot be bothered to improve his technique it is important that the woman grasps the underlying message (that is, he does not care enough about the relationship or her to work on it). How each individual chooses to deal with the situation is beyond the scope of this book but, obviously, a partner has to ask herself if it is worth prolonging such a relationship.

Anxiety, fear and inhibition

These may also freeze sexual arousal. If this is the case it is important to examine what has led you to have such fears in the first place. Delving into your background, your upbringing and your past relationships with men is a way of doing this. Women's sexuality groups offer a powerfully effective way of doing this in a supportive atmosphere and offer, by virtue of the group's participation in your problems, several alternative perspectives. Assertion groups offer something similar with a specific teaching in how to be less afraid when attempting to 'be yourself'. Personal counselling helps you examine fears and assists you to work out your own methods of dealing with them. Co-counselling, which is a do-it-yourself method of personal counselling, offers the same. Co-counselling consists of getting together with a friend or acquaintance, solely for the purpose of discussing personal problems and working out solutions. Each partner takes it in turns. The first hour is spent solely on the one partner, the second on the other partner. Simple rules are used such as not putting forward your own opinions if you are the listener but merely asking 'What does that make you feel?' 'What do you think about this?' The main purpose is to get the person revealing to concentrate on their own feelings and not those of anyone else in their life. For both personal counselling and co-counselling to work well there needs to be an agreement to meet regularly over a long period of time—at least six months.

Lack of attraction or affection, towards a partner

These may also be culprits. Here it is the relationship itself which needs consideration. Does the lack of attraction mean there is a lack of love? Is there some traumatic hangover from previous experiences which is being transferred to the present relationship? Is the relationship continuing for reasons other than sexuality? If the problem involves a long-term partnership where, for example, a family makes it desirable to remain together, does the solution to the sexual difficulty lie with someone outside the marriage? These are all questions which could healthily be debated by couples wanting to improve their sex lives without the aid of a therapist.

According to Dr Helen Singer Kaplan, the outcome for couples who lack desire for each other is not very good. She estimates that a mere 15 to 20 per cent are likely to regain sexual desire for each other as the result of therapy (see Chapter 2). However, couple therapy with a sex therapist is one way in which to resolve some of the marital problems which can result in painful intercourse. See Chapter 2 for more details.

Menopause

Women who have gone through the menopause may produce less lubrication than formerly owing to hormone changes. But if this causes pain the GP can prescribe hormone replacement therapy which puts oestrogen, and therefore moistness, back into the vaginal tissue. See Chapter 7 for more details.

Vaginal problems

Vaginal infections

One of the most usual causes of painful intercourse is vaginal infection, the most common being *monilia* or *thrush* (for details on what causes this and how to deal with it, see Chapter 5 on Sexual Health). Another common infection is *trichomoniasis* (also see Chapter 5).

A variety of bacteria can affect the vagina and if bacterial infections are persistent, the personal hygiene of *both* partners should be investigated, with special attention to the role of anal sex. If a couple has *anal intercourse* prior to vaginal intercourse, bacteria is spread very easily. The solution is never to have anal intercourse first.

Herpes virus and warts virus, where they infect the interior of the genitals and are not visible on the outside can also cause pain (see Chapter 5).

Vaginal allergies

Very occasionally the sensitive vaginal membrane becomes allergic.
- Rubber contraception is one offender
- Chemical contraception is another
- Vaginal deodorants can also cause problems. The solution is to avoid the offending substances.
- Very rarely, a woman is allergic to her partner's sperm but the use of condoms usually helps prevent an allergic reaction.

Vaginal size

Sometimes partners believe that the female vagina is too small to accommodate the penis but in fact, this is rarely the case. The vagina is capable of dilating very widely indeed—look how it has to stretch during childbirth, for example. So, the only real problem to arise would be if you possessed a particularly tough hymen which refused to break as a result of the normal thrusting of the penis or finger dilation. Simple medical help solves this problem—the GP can break the hymen for you surgically while using a local anaesthetic.

Occasionally, during first and early intercourse, the tender vaginal skin may sustain minor cuts or bruises, causing temporary discomfort. But these abrasions, if left undisturbed for a short time, will heal rapidly by themselves.

Penis size

Very rarely, penis size may be at fault: a few (very few) men possess abnormally large penises. Contrary to myth, these can cause bruising and pain rather than raptures of delight, and less boisterous types of intercourse may need to be practised.

Internal pain

Childbirth, abortion or accidents may produce scarring on the walls of the vagina. These scars, when stretched during intercourse, can be painful and episiotomy scars, for example, commonly upset intercourse. Usually these become more flexible with time and the pain fades but, occasionally, the episiotomy has been so badly sutured that the scarring is very wide indeed. The best solution here is to ask for minor vaginal surgery, where the episiotomy is reopened, the scar tissue excised and the cut correctly stitched up. Where surgery is not called for but nevertheless there is persistent pain during certain sexual positions, the solution is to work out alternative positions where the tender spots are not stretched so drastically. If, for example, there is scarring on the left side of the vagina, missionary position intercourse can be modified to take place on the other side. If you lie on the side which is painful (the left side) the penis (also approaching from the side) is likely to penetrate in the direction of the right vaginal wall and thus, hopefully, will avoid creating discomfort.

Gynaecological illness

Ovarian cysts, tubal infections, pelvic inflammatory disease and endometriosis

These can all cause extreme discomfort when the penis thrusts towards the affected area. Medical aid must be sought for these conditions since antibiotic treatment and in some cases surgery is indicated.

Displacement of the uterus

One of the most common causes of pain is displacement of the uterus during penetration. The uterus is attached to the pelvic cavity by ligaments and it is their flexibility which allows the uterus to move around in a limited way. The ligaments are themselves endowed with nerve endings. During certain positions of intercourse, the uterus—where it projects into the upper vagina—comes directly into line with the penis. When this happens, the penis, during thrusting, pushes the uterus up towards the abdomen, at the same time stretching the ligaments uncomfortably and provoking their nerve endings to give a painful reaction.

The most common positions to cause this are those where deep thrusting is enjoyed—for example:

- In the male superior position where the woman's legs are over the man's shoulders or wrapped around his waist
- Or where the woman sits astride the man in a kneeling position, her legs on either side of his body.

This pain is usually felt in the lower part of the uterus and around the cervix, but it does not mean that there is anything physically wrong. It simply means that the woman cannot tolerate the sensation of her womb being pushed too far from its normal position.

The solution is not instantly to give up favourite sex positions—although choosing others would, of course, alleviate the problem. It is rather to make readjustments. In the case of the male superior position mentioned, it is possible either for the woman to twist her pelvis a little or, to lie across the bed (on her back) with her legs over the sides while her partner kneels or stands on the floor. This allows him more easily to alter the angle of his thrust away from the cervix while still giving the sensation of deep thrusting. If *all* front position intercourse results in pain, vaginal rear entry may be a more comfortable alternative.

In the case of the woman astride position, if the woman arches away from the man's body as she thrusts, or lies forward along his body, or simply bends one knee more than the other so that her pelvis is tilted differently, she is likely to avoid hard contact with the uterus and instead, direct the penis into other areas of the vagina. Just alter the angle of thrust and you avoid pain!

Hysterectomy

Some women experience pain as a result of hysterectomy (removal of the womb). In some cases the pain has psychological causes and results from inadequate explanations of what the surgery entailed or from fears about intercourse after the operation. Careful explanation of the operation, reassurance and lovemaking which includes a lot of manual love-play and little intercourse should aid recovery.

Physical causes of painful intercourse after hysterectomy include stitches or scar tissue which the penis hits. Alternative positions should be used until the tissue has healed.

Women who have had their ovaries removed at the same time as the hysterectomy and who haven't been given hormone replacement therapy may experience a drying-up of vaginal lubrication and therefore increasingly sensitive vaginal tissue. By going onto hormone replacement (which helps keep the tissue soft) the soreness and discomfort dissipates.

Pelvic congestion

Just like men who are sexually stimulated but unable to reach orgasm suffer from the colloquially named 'balls-ache', so too do women experience a similar condition. Called *pelvic congestion*, it consists of a dull-throbbing, menstrual-type pain, deep in the pelvis. It can last for some hours and in extreme cases for a couple of days. The antidote is an orgasm—and if a woman is unable to experience orgasm during intercourse she would be wise to give herself one with masturbation or ask her partner to do so.

Orgasmic pain

Ironically, perhaps, in the light of the above advice a very few women experience pain *during or after orgasm*. Usually this is a result of very strong or prolonged orgasm, or often thanks to multi-orgasmic activity. There is unlikely to be anything physically wrong. The vaginal muscles may simply be asking for a period of rest. Vaginal muscles can be strained by over-activity, just as any other.

Vaginismus

Vaginismus is a relatively rare disorder in which involuntary tensing of the vagina sends it into spasms. This makes vaginal penetration impossible or at the very least, extremely difficult.

Vaginismus happens unconsciously as the result of some kind of past shock or physically painful event. It is a self-imposed conditioning based on the memories of such an event. Perhaps there was a sexual assault when young, a painful vaginal experience half-forgotten, physical disease, conscious or unconscious fears. Sometimes the traumatic cause is forgotten or just cannot be identified, but the spasms are still there.

The problem usually becomes apparent during first or early lovemaking but occasionally it prevents teenagers from using tampons when they menstruate. Some women find they also tense up deeply in the GP's surgery, making vaginal examination impossible.

Treatment This consists mainly of eliminating the conditioned response (spasm) by teaching the sufferer to insert small and then increasingly larger phallic-shaped objects into her vagina. This very simple method teaches tolerance of penetration but it is sometimes necessary to examine what caused the spasmic reflex in the first place. For example, fear of penetration may be accompanied by phobic feelings about intercourse and about the men who want intercourse. These fears are often experienced only subconsciously and may need to be drawn out so that they can be examined and the emotional responses reworked.

Self-help therapy (over 14 days) When the traumatic causes are understood or at least while they are being explored you are asked to examine your vagina in a mirror when you are on your own, in the privacy of your home. You are asked to place your index finger at the entrance to your vagina and see what it feels like to insert the finger tip. These feelings can be discussed with your partner at a later date.

When you have been able to insert a fingertip, you are next asked to insert the whole finger. Then two fingers. All fears and anxieties thrown up now or during any of the process need to be talked about with your partner afterwards.

Next you are asked to insert a tampon (leaving its lubricated cardboard cover on) and to leave it there for several hours or until it feels completely comfortable. You may feel some anxiety and tightness when you do this but not pain. Naturally you are expected to remain resting—in a reclining, not sitting position—perhaps reading, during this session. (You are *not* supposed to walk around with the tampon inside you.) The tightness and anxiety will not increase, and if you tolerate the tampon and its casing inside you for a little while, the feelings of tension will begin to dissipate. The next time you use the tampon you are encouraged to do so for a little longer until finally you feel comfortable and *in control* during this type of penetration.

At the next stage your partner is involved. He is asked to look carefully at your vagina, then asked to repeat the procedure that you have so far carried out on yourself. First he inserts a fingertip into your vagina. Then, while you guide and control his hand, he slips the whole finger in. To begin with, he holds it there quietly while you learn to contain it, just as you did with the tampon. In the next stage he moves the finger gently in and out of the vagina with your hand still guiding him. Then he tries two fingers. During this entire phase both of you remain aware of the fact that whatever happens, *there will be no penile penetration.* It is at this stage that the procedure often stops being technical and becomes sexual. Once the woman feels relaxed and no longer fears the penetrating finger she may easily become aroused.

The first penetration of the penis is, of course, important. The event is agreed on beforehand and your partner lubricates his penis and penetrates with the help of your guiding hand. He remains quietly within your vagina for a few minutes without thrusting so that you learn to relax and contain him. Then he withdraws. Whether or not you both choose to continue that lovemaking session without a second penetration is, of course, entirely your own choice.

At the next session penetration is followed by resting still within the vagina for a short time and then making some gentle thrusting. Subsequent sessions can take penetration and thrusting further until such a time as they culminate in orgasm.

Perhaps the most difficult time during this whole 'home-practice' procedure is that leading up to and just before the penetration of the penis. After penetration, there is a marked gain in self-confidence when the woman realizes she has overcome her tense feelings.

Providing the moves are taken slowly and carefully, with adequate discussion at the appropriate times, this is successful for the majority of couples. Occasionally self-help shows that there are other sexual dysfunctions getting in the way of good sex and if this is the case, further help should be sought from a sex therapist.

If self-help of this kind *without* the aid of a therapist is not successful, there is still a strong likelihood that the same methods, but with the support of a therapist, *will* work.

Sudden change

When a couple who have previously enjoyed blissfully satisfying pain-free sex for years suddenly develop problems and all the physical causes described in this chapter have been investigated, it is worth finding out if anything else in their sex life has changed recently.

Dr Jules Black, a consultant gynaecologist from Australia, tells an amusing tale of a couple in this category. He tracked the cause of their problems down to their new water bed. Because the bed was constantly 'on the move' the couple were finding that intercourse was hitting parts hitherto unreached, slamming the penis randomly into the uterus as described earlier. The bed, alas, had to go!

Physical pain during intercourse can disrupt the most delightful relationship. No man likes to think that every time he feels sexy he will cause his loved one pain. No woman wants to anticipate sexual agony on a regular basis. So if your love-making stops for these reasons, your doctor should be consulted as soon as possible.

PART 2

Sexual Health Problems

FIVE

Sexual Diseases

Special clinics (VD clinics) have observed that as many as one quarter of the people attending, have sex problems. The link between sex problems and STD (sexually transmitted disease) is unspecified but, as we have already seen in Chapter 5, on painful sex, certain vaginal conditions such as thrush or herpes can make sex a painful experience and set up tensions which affect the quality of intercourse.

At present there is a tendency to use fewer barrier methods of contraception (the pill is usually first choice) so we have less protection from sexually transmitted disease. Also, we are starting our sex lives earlier than former generations have done and the available evidence indicates that this increases the likelihood of sexual disease.

New knowledge about the womb lining of early teenage women shows it is not always mature enough to cope with organisms that are introduced during intercourse. The majority of STD specialists think that this leads to an increased likelihood of cellular changes within the vaginal tissues which, if untreated, may become cancerous. Postponing first experiences of intercourse until late teenage and returning to the more 'old-fashioned' methods of contraception (such as the diaphragm or sheath) are the obvious methods of safeguarding sexual health in the early years.

There has been much debate about the role that the male foreskin plays in women's genital health and there is increasing evidence to show that if the foreskin harbours bacteria this can trigger off infections in the woman—most noticeably thrush. The 'ping-pong' syndrome in which partners constantly re-infect each other is a distressing example of cross-transmission. There have also been cases where herpes sores are concealed by the foreskin and only discovered after the woman has developed the virus.

The moral of this is to ensure before intercourse that your partner's genitals are clean and healthy or, at least, that a condom is worn. Very young women should also bear in mind that good sex doesn't have to include intercourse. There are other sexual activities two people can enjoy.

Not all the responsibility for sexual health lies with the man. Just because half the female genitalia lies hidden within the body, does not mean that hygiene can be neglected. By regularly inspecting the genitals with the aid of a mirror and by using a transparent speculum—a polished instrument designed to help you to view the insides of the vagina and the cervix—you can learn what is normal for this part of your anatomy and what is not. If a problematic discharge or condition of the cervix is spotted early on, medical help can be sought earlier, the condition cleared up quickly and the likelihood of the condition being spread lessened. Cheap disposable plastic speculae can be bought from large chemists and surgical suppliers. (For details on how to use them see Appendix 1 on p. 171).

The rest of this chapter describes the main sexual diseases and ailments in alphabetical order. There is a section on VD clinics at the end of the chapter.

AIDS (Acquired Immuno Deficiency Syndrome)

Many people erroneously believe that AIDS is a disease confined to homosexual men. While this is mainly true in the Western world it is important to understand that women can and do catch it also. At present, Western women are in a lesser risk category than men, while lesbians are in the lowest risk category of all.

Aids isn't something you catch like 'flu. It is, in fact, a syndrome that develops after catching another virus, HTLV3. If you come into contact with HTLV3 you are likely (but it is not certain) to develop antibodies to the virus. These can be detected by a test, but all they prove is that you have been in touch with the virus and you are said to be 'antibody positive'. This does not necessarily mean you are infectious. At present it cannot be shown whether people with HTLV3 antibodies are infectious or not, although it would be wise to take precautions in the event of your partner being antibody positive or, indeed, if you are the one in that situation. The best precaution is, of course, to avoid having sex again! A rather more realistic one is to confine yourself to a single partner.

Around 10 per cent of such people may go on to develop symptoms of AIDS with either minor or severe symptoms.

Treatment While symptoms, even when severe, may be effectively treated, there is as yet no way of eliminating the virus because the HTLV3 virus makes the 'helper' cells in our body vulnerable to cancer, pneumonia and other hazards of the environment. In America, the Centre of Disease Control has reported 8,597 cases; of those 4,145 are dead. What is more, the number of cases is doubling every 14 months. In England, there were 140 cases reported in early 1985 with 62 dead and the number is doubling every six months.

We are in the early stages of understanding this disease. Nobody can say for sure what future course the disease will follow. Or exactly how many men and women who come into contact with HTLV3 will suffer a breakdown of their immune system. It is alleged that in certain African countries many women have AIDS as well as their partners. It has also been shown that 40 per cent of women prostitutes in one large American city are antibody positive, and this is likely to become the case in the UK.

The likelihood of contracting HTLV3 through anything other than intimate sexual or blood contact is virtually nil. There is no documented case of the virus being spread by saliva. The element of risk of catching HTLV3 from an infected partner is reckoned to be 50 per cent. Bisexuals are particularly likely to spread the disease and in America the number of women believed to have contracted HTLV3 from bisexual lovers is assessed at 62.

People who receive blood transfusions in this country were at some risk since the disease can be transferred through blood, but since October 1985 all donated blood used in the UK is given a heat treatment which removes the virus if it exists.

Exactly how the disease is transferred during sexual intercourse is uncertain but one theory is that it might be passed on through an open cut or tear in the body via semen. While research work to understand the illness better and to develop an anti-viral drug or vaccine is progressing rapidly, the best way at present to contain the disease is to appeal for co-operation from men and women in altering their sexual lifestyle. Many homosexual men are abandoning certain sex acts, including anal intercourse and love-biting. If women suspect that their partner might be a high risk HTLV3 carrier because he is known to be bisexual, they would be wise to refrain from these activities too.

In England a trust has been created to help people with fears about AIDS and to provide support. (The Terence Higgins Trust. Tel: 01–833 2971.)

Crabs or pubic lice

'Crabs' are tiny crab-shaped lice which live in pubic hair (they occasionally spread to other body hair). They are caught by sexual contact (whether or not intercourse is involved) or from bedding, someone else's clothes or towels. You usually discover you have crabs when acute itching develops in your pubic area. Although tiny, it is possible to see the egg cases or 'nits' at the base of the pubic hair.

Treatment A shampoo called Lorexane or Quellada (available from any chemist) or free from a special clinic, i.e. the genito-urinary or VD clinic at your nearest big hospital, will eradicate the lice within twenty-four hours. Dramatic methods such as dowsing yourself with Dettol should *not* be used, since these don't clear up the lice and they do inflict chemical burns if used neat. It is advisable that your partner similarly uses the shampoo and you should avoid suspect bedding etc. Although the crabs die within twenty-four hours, their eggs live for about six days and it is wise therefore to re-shampoo a week later.

Cystitis

Cystitis is a condition of the bladder and is an 'umbrella' term used to describe various unexplained infections or bladder problems. The symptoms of true cystitis, however, are:
● pain and increased frequency of urination
● sometimes blood loss from the urethra while urinating.

It is caused by bruising or infection and is nicknamed the 'honeymooner's disease' because so many young brides experience cystitis for the first time on their honeymoon. The infection may already be present within the body in the kidneys or the bloodstream and *descends* to the urethra to cause the symptoms, or it may be introduced from outside the body (such as from a partner) and in this case it *a*scends to the urethra.

Frequent and enthusiastic intercourse can bruise the cervix, opening it up to infection. E-coli (escherichia coli) is the main germ responsible for the infection since this normally lives in the bowel and may be transferred easily. E-coli may also be situated beneath the partner's foreskin and the condition can sometimes 'ping-pong'. Poor hygiene is often responsible for such germs and, unromantic though it may sound, a good wash before and after intercourse can be a sensible preventative measure.

Intercourse experienced when there is little vaginal lubrication can cause dry internal tissue to split and provide a site for infection.

Anything that affects the acid-alkaline balance of the vagina can predispose a woman to cystitis:
- Hormone changes
- Foaming contraceptives, pessaries and the pill
- Damage as a result of childbirth
- Kidney problems (children who hold their urine instead of asking to leave the room may bruise themselves internally and develop the problem)
- Antibiotics
- Growths in the renal channels or in the bladder
- Diabetes, pre-diabetes and kidney stones.

Treatment. If left untreated cystitis can develop into serious and painful kidney infections. It is important, therefore, that an attack is dealt with as rapidly as possible. The Health Education Council, in association with Angela Kilmartin (a pioneer of cystitis self-help), have developed the following self-help measures to be started as soon as an attack is apparent.
1   Pass a specimen into a clean jar for analysis by your GP.
2   Immediately drink one pint of cold water.
3   After letting your stomach settle a little, add a teaspoon of bicarbonate of soda to some water or diluted fruit squash and drink. Repeat this twice more at hourly intervals. (Heart patients *must* discuss taking bicarbonate with their doctors first.)
4   Drink half a pint of liquid (weak tea, dilute squash or, best of all, plain water) every 20 minutes.

5   Painkillers (preferably not aspirin) can deaden the pain.
6   A cup of strong black coffee every hour will make sure you
expel the liquid you are taking in.
7   While you are doing all this, between trips to the loo, you
should be resting close by. Sit with your feet up and a hot-water
bottle between your legs, with others behind your back and
against your stomach.

If you adhere faithfully to the above routine the germs should
be flushed out of your system within three hours. The earlier
you get to grips with the symptoms, the more rapidly you are
likely to quell the attack. Don't worry if, for the first half an
hour, the attack worsens. This is because the high intake of
liquid hasn't yet had time to reach the urethra and start
flushing. Continue with the routine.

Cystitis and sex

The implications cystitis holds for a sex life are obvious. A mild
bout means sex is merely uncomfortable, while a bout in full
spate means sex becomes impossible. Continual recurring
bouts of cystitis which are not quickly dealt with can make a
regular sex life extremely difficult to attain and in severe cases
can even break up a marriage. It is important for male partners
to check the bacterial condition of their own sexual organ and to
employ the best possible measures of hygiene. Men, while
possessing their own urethral problems, rarely get cystitis, but
they can harbour E-coli.

Cytomegalovirus

This is a rare virus which causes debilitating illness similar to
glandular fever and can be spread by kissing and sexual
intercourse. It is potentially extremely damaging to the
developing foetus and babies can be born with deafness,
blindness or even spastic paralysis as a result. Most people
affected show no symptoms of the virus at all and it doesn't
cause them any long-term damage. It doesn't therefore immediately affect the sex life but all potential mothers are
automatically given tests to discover whether or not they have

the virus. If there is any reason to think cytomegalovirus may affect you, you should seek medical advice.

Gardnerella vaginalis

Gardnerella vaginalis is the second most common cause of vaginal discharge. It is characterized by a smelly greyish-white, non-irritating fluid which contains gardnerella bacteria. This discharge was categorized for years as one of the causes of NSU (non-specific urethritis) but has now been identified as a quite separate organism. Since the discharge is similar it is often diagnozed as trichomoniasis, but it is in fact a bacteria while 'trich' is a parasite. However, the same drug treatment wipes both out; that is Flagyl.

One of the problems with gardnerella is that it is difficult to identify. Time and again women leave the surgery or special clinic with the information that tests have proved to be negative and therefore there is nothing wrong with them. But it is *not normal* continually to produce a strong-smelling discharge. It is uncertain at present whether this is sexually transmitted, although it seems highly likely. There is also a possibility that it might be introduced by sources such as tampons.

Genital warts

Genital warts are caused by a virus very similar to that of warts situated on other parts of the body. They are sexually transmitted and in general grow to a larger size than do warts which are non-genital. Up till recently they have been thought to be as harmless as the ordinary variety but new research shows that the sexually transmitted type is implicated in cervical cancer.

The warts appear usually about three months to a year after sexual contact with an infected partner. When small they resemble ordinary but pointed warts. When larger they assume a cauliflower-like shape. They tend to proliferate during pregnancy but naturally regress once pregnancy has ended.

As with ordinary warts virus, the warts may recur at intervals of stress but eventually regress with the passage of time. Genital warts are situated on or inside the vagina and the anus, although rarely they appear in the mouth when the sufferer has caught them from oral sex. In women they are often accompanied by a vaginal discharge which also needs to be treated. Men usually get warts under the foreskin, although they can also be sited on the shaft of the penis and on the glans.

Treatment It is important to try and eradicate all the warts in one go because if any are left they spread and reoccupy the former site. If the warts are small they can be dried up with an application of podophyllin, an ointment or liquid which can be obtained on prescription. This is left on the skin for four hours and then washed off to avoid 'burning' the area. If it is necessary to repeat the treatment this must be done under medical supervision as too frequent exposures to the medication can harm the sensitive vaginal tissue.

If the warts are not eradicated this way or if they are too large to respond to such treatment, they can be treated with cryosurgery (freezing them off) or burnt off with electrocautery. Podophyllin should *not* be used during pregnancy. Sexual partners should also be examined and treated.

Other effects of warts. Large outcrops of warts on the genitals are hardly conducive to a relaxed sex life. Even though they do not hurt, their shape and bulk may deter your partner from sex. Rapid recognition of the condition and equally rapid treatment is the best way of dealing with it. The less time it is given to interefere with your sex life, the better.

Since cellular changes in the cervix have now been associated with the warts virus, if you know you have the condition you would be wise to seek a six-monthly cervical smear, either on the National Health or privately.

Gonorrhoea

Gonorrhoea generally responds well to certain antibiotics and, although most women show no visible sign of the bacteria, they should always seek examination if they know their partner has it. If left untreated, gonorrhoea can cause salpingitis (a painful inflammation of the Fallopian tubes) and sterility and peritonitis (rupture of the abdominal wall) which is potentially fatal.

In men the signs are a thick milky discharge and a burning

sensation while urinating. Women may develop a cervical discharge. Female symptoms develop anything from two days to three weeks after contact with an infected partner and forty to fifty per cent of women in contact go on to develop the disease. It is also possible to spread it by methods other than sexual intercourse, including the hands and the mouth. Lesbian couples are just as vulnerable as heterosexual ones. For women on the pill the risks of developing the illness are higher, since the pill does not provide a barrier protection for the cervix and uterus as does the sheath and diaphragm and the spread of infection seems to be more rapid.

Treatment A high dosage of penicillin usually clears up the condition. It is important to trace all sexual contacts and to return to the clinic for follow-up checks to make quite sure that the infection has been eradicated.

It is also worth noting that barrier methods of contraception, such as the sheath or diaphragm used with Ortho-Gynol Jelly or Ortho Cream, have been shown to lessen the likelihood of developing the disease after sexual contact.

Children born to women with gonorrhoea must have their eyes treated with silver nitrate or penicillin drops to prevent gonoccocal conjunctivitis.

Herpes genitalis

One estimate of the growth of herpes reckons that it increases by ten per cent every year. However, there has been so much published on the subject that this has undoubtedly affected sexual behaviour in the same way that the AIDs scare is presently doing. People with formerly promiscuous lifestyles are now confining their lovemaking to a regular partner or within a regular group. Herpes self-help groups are springing up which promote friendships among herpes sufferers so that any stigma can be discussed and dealt with and so that the herpes is contained within the group rather than allowed to put other people at risk.

Herpes is a virus which can attack men and women alike. The genital variety is called herpes simplex 2 and the old-fashioned, cold-sore-around-the-mouth type is herpes simplex 1. The two types are related and can cross over if the partners involved practise oral sex. The treatment of both types on the genitals is similar.

Herpes simplex 2 is sexually transmitted and appears as small blisters. In women these blisters—which eventually become open sores—may be situated on the cervix, vagina, labia, thighs, in or near the anus and the buttocks. When they are open sores they are highly contagious. An attack may last for anything from a week to a month before the sores heal and finally disappear. The virus, however, remains dormant within the spinal column and at times of stress is likely to recur. The estimate of recurrence is anything from forty to seventy per cent. While some people suffer acutely from the condition and develop other associated infections and fevers it has to be stressed that these sufferers are a small minority. The majority of people get the condition mildly and it is estimated that about half the people who get the genital version of herpes don't even know they have had it.

Treatment. As yet, there are no known cures which eliminate the virus from the sufferer's body. However, there is a great deal of viral research at present aiming at elimination. An important drug called acylovir (Zovirax) has been available for the past few years which lessens the effects of the attacks when they do occur and lessen the numbers and strength of future attacks. Since it is stress which triggers off further attacks—at the risk of sounding simplistic—avoiding stress is one way of avoiding more herpes.

Other effects of herpes. The impact of herpes on your sex life depends largely on the amount of anxiety it creates. Some people are able to continue with their love life with no apparent trauma, while others sense the stigma keenly and feel they are not worthy of any relationships at all. Since it is inadvisable to have intercourse during the open sores stage, this naturally limits sexual relationships although there is no reason why other loving contact cannot be substituted temporarily. Acute cases, where the herpes causes great pain, can however destroy relationships and put the sufferer through mental agony.

Herpes is likely to have more impact on your love life if you are unattached, rather than if you are already in an established relationship, and the knowledge that every new friendship must necessarily be preceded with a confession which might not be accepted with enthusiasm can be very depressing. The self-help solution, which is to find your partners among the already afflicted, may be one way of dealing with this.

Dangerous side-effects include the possible infection of a baby, if born when its mother is having an active attack. To avoid this likelihood (which can cause brain damage in the baby or even kill it) all mothers with active herpes at the time of delivery are advised to have their babies by caesarian section.

Cancer of the cervix in some women is now also associated with herpes genitalis. In practical terms this means that once you know you have the condition you would be wise to get a regular cervical smear *once every six months* even if you cannot do so on the National Health Service and therefore have to pay for it to be done privately.

NSU (Non specific urethritis)

This condition is much more serious for men than it is for women and, in rare cases, leads to Reiter's syndrome. This is a crippling form of arthritis. However, women should not ignore NSU since they may be carriers and therefore re-infect their partners. Women can also get Reiter's syndrome, but there is less likelihood of this happening.

NSU organisms produce a whitish discharge and cervicitis although some women may have the condition and be quite unaware of it. NSU is also sometimes associated with bouts of eye infection ('red eye') and occasionally with trichomoniasis. (see p. 75 for more details.)

Treatment. The treatment for NSU is tetracycline, during which time the patient is advised to abstain from intercourse and alcohol.

PID (Pelvic inflammatory disease)

This disease consists of a variety of pelvic infections which affect the uterus (parametritis), the tubes (salpingitis), and the tubes and ovaries (salpingo-oophoritis). It can be caused by bacteria, certain viruses or gonorrhoea.

The infections may be caused via sexual intercourse—although this is not always the case. Women with IUDs are specially prone to PID.

PID symptoms include:

- A tender or painful abdomen
- Pain on intercourse or menstruation
- Irregular bleeding
- Occasional chills and fevers.

The disease can produce scarring of the Fallopian tubes and if allowed to continue can cause sterility by eventually blocking the tubes with scar tissue. It is wise therefore to take any symptoms to the doctor as soon as possible.

Treatment Treatment consists of tetracycline or ampicillin, bed rest if the condition is severe and no sexual intercourse for at least two weeks in order to give the infected area time in which to recover. Women who have had PID are specially prone to ectopic pregnancies (that is, where the fertilized egg lies in one of the Fallopian tubes or in the abdominal cavity, and not in the womb).

The side-effects of pain on a sex life are examined in detail in Chapter 4 but it is important to make it clear to partners that the pain experienced is real, that it can be cleared up with the right treatment and that meanwhile patience needs to be exercised in a good cause!

Syphilis

In the last two decades syphilis has remained at a constantly low level, thanks to the efficacy of penicillin and to the routine checks that every pregnant woman receives in early ante-natal care to ascertain whether or not she may have the disease. In 1984 only 2,933 cases were reported in the UK.

However, the final stages of syphilis can deform, lead to madness and even death, not to mention passing the same problems on to your children, so it is worth being aware of the symptoms.

Primary syphilis

Women are frequently unaware that they have syphilis since the syphilitic ulcer may be sited inside the vagina. However, it can also develop on the labia, the clitoris or the urethra.

Male partners find that the painless sore or ulcer appears on the glans (head of the penis), the shaft, and the scrotum. It may sometimes be hidden beneath the foreskin or be sited directly underneath the scrotum or where the penis meets the body. The ulcer is absolutely painless and takes anything from nine to ninety days to appear after contact with a syphilitic partner. The primary chancre, as it was traditionally called, may be pimple-sized and looks like a blister or an open sore. If left completely alone the sore goes away by itself within one to five weeks, but the bacteria responsible remains within the body and eventually leads to a later stage of syphilis. It is at this stage of the disease that syphilis is highly contagious. Contact with any open sore and even kissing can spread the organism.

Secondary syphilis

The second stage occurs anything from a week to six months later.
- There is a generalized itchy rash on the genitals and, in some cases over the entire body.
- Sores may occur in the mouth.
- The lymph glands around the genital area may become enlarged and painful.
- Joints may become swollen and painful.
- There may be flu-like symptoms.
- Patches of hair may fall out.

Sometimes the secondary stage is so mild, however, that none of these symptoms are noticed. In either case, if left untreated the secondary symptoms also disappear from two to six weeks after their first appearance. But again the organisms are left within the body. After that the infection is more likely to be diagnozed by blood tests and is described as latent.

Latent syphilis

The latent stage can last for ten or even twenty years but, during this time, the organism is attacking the body internally. After about a year of the latent stage the sufferer ceases to be infectious—except in the case of pregnancy where the unborn child may develop congenital syphilis caught from the mother. The last stage of the disease (which appears only during middle age) can involve any part of the body but particularly attacks the brain. This eventually proves fatal.

It must be stressed that with present medical diagnosis and drug treatment syphilis should never be allowed to reach this stage, and it is indeed extremely rare. Primary and secondary syphilis can be treated with penicillin. Latent syphilis also responds to penicillin and prevents the internal damage from going any further. What it can't do, of course, is restore the organs to their former full working order.

Thrush (candida albicans)

Thrush shows as a white coating on the walls of the vagina. It frequently produces a discharge that resembles cottage cheese and has a rich, yeasty smell. The condition can be irritating and scratching exacerbates it.

Extreme cases of thrush are so painful that sex is prohibited and even less extreme cases can make sex so uncomfortable that many thoughts of sexual pleasure are lost. Since some women appear to have a greater tendency to suffer from thrush than others, prevention is just as important as cure.

The circulation of air around the genitals allows the area to dry out and become less attractive for the thrush fungus. This means that nylon tights, nylon panties and tight, heavy jeans should not be worn. Cotton underwear and tights with a cotton gusset or no tights at all are preferable.

Too much sugar in the diet can promote the growth of thrush, so it helps if sugar is cut out. Diabetics are particularly prone to thrush thanks to their 'sugar problem' and women with recurrent thrush would do well to seek medical examination for a possible diabetic condition. It is important to remember that many prepared foods contain sugar: tomato ketchup and sweet pickles, for example, contain a lot.

Further causes include antibiotics, hormonal changes (i.e., going on to the pill), swimming in crowded public pools, sitting all day long on a nylon-covered seat, pregnancy.

Partners may harbour thrush spores although they may not realize this. If you are being treated for recurring thrush you should also obtain medication for your partner. This includes lesbian women.

Prevention If antibiotics for some other condition are essential, ask the doctor for a nystatin prescription at the same time. Banish sugar from your diet, cut down alcohol, avoid hot baths and have showers instead if you can. Keep a special flannel for the genitals only and boil this cloth every other day. Avoid swimming in public pools. Choose a method of contraception other than the pill. And never wear nylon tights—especially when taking part in a sporting activity.

Treatment A variety of drugs are effective in clearing up thrush. These include nystatin (Nystan), clotromazole (Canestan), miconazole nitrate (Gyno-Daktarin, Monistat). While these are equally efficient in eliminating thrush, trials show that women suffer from fewer recurring bouts when using miconazole nitrate. The same drug treatment should be used by your partner. These substances are mainly available as ointments but are sometimes also provided in pill form.

Self-help methods of cure include inserting a little live yogurt into the vagina (use a small, plastic squeeze bottle for this purpose) and then keep the yoghurt in place with a tampon. Or use Lactic pessaries (obtainable from some chemists) which alter the acidity of the vaginal secretion, and make the vaginal conditions unpleasant for the thrush.

Trichomoniasis

For women, this is the third most common sexually transmitted problem and is easily identifiable by the appalling smell of the thin yellow discharge which can make the inside and outside of the vagina red and sore. There is also increased frequency of urination accompanied by a painful, burning sensation each time. Trichomonas vaginalis is a one-celled parasite found in men and women but most commonly with men, there are no obvious symptoms.

Trichomoniasis is usually spread by sexual transmission but can also be transferred from shared towels, from toilet paper or the toilet seat.

Treatment Flagyl will clear up the condition but must not be taken during pregnancy, or if you are possibly pregnant (it can affect the embryo) or if you are breastfeeding. Ask the GP for alternative treatment. Also, Flagyl should be taken with meals as it can otherwise irritate the throat. If combined with alcohol, it can cause nausea.

VD clinics

Although many individual GPs may be experienced in successfully diagnosing sexually transmitted diseases it is, in general, a greater safeguard for your personal health to bring problems of sexual health to the nearest venereal or special clinic. Since these clinics specialize in sexually transmitted disease, they are expert at diagnosing and treating them.

Special or VD clinics are mainly found in big teaching hospitals. They practise strict anonymity, identifying patients by numbers rather than names. The stigma of attending a VD clinic has lessened considerably in the past few years since the majority of women patients attending do so because thrush (monilia or candida—not always sexually transmitted) is the main cause of complaint. As the venereal consultant at Westminster Hospital is famous for once having said, 'some of the nicest people are my patients'.

Unlike most hospital departments patients can refer themselves to a Special clinic. They do not need a doctor's letter but it is advisable to book an appointment by telephone as clinic time is not always available to drop-in patients.

A first visit usually includes diagnosis and treatment. But if diagnosis can't be done instantly a further visit may be necessary, to hear the results of tests and to receive treatment. A further follow-up is *always* required to make certain the treatment has worked and you will usually be asked whom were your sexual contacts. Many special clinics employ contact tracers who are responsible for finding men and women who could also be at risk as a result of your relationship with them. If the problem recurs, your regular partner should be asked to attend for treatment too.

If you do not hear any news after tests have been made *do not assume all is well*. Telephone the clinic and insist they check they have received the results of the tests and insist that they tell you what these are. Hospitals and GPs have been known to overlook test results through overwork or forgetfulness. If the tests have been positive ones, obviously, such an oversight could be very serious indeed—for you.

If, at any stage of treatment at the Special clinic, a patient feels seriously dissatisfied with the standard of treatment, they are entitled to lodge a complaint with the consultant. Such complaints usually ensure that the patient is taken seriously.

VD clinics are situated in most major hospitals and the telephone numbers of these can be found in the telephone directory either under the individual name of the hospital or under a main heading HOSPITAL.

SIX

Hormones and Sex

How hormones function within us is a complex and still only partially understood subject. Each hormone within the body exerts a subtle influence on the others and if one somehow becomes 'out of sync' the others may also go through changes in order to compensate.

Hormones related to sexual function

Although many hormones exercise their function within our blood chemistry there are three sets of sex steroids which are principally associated with sexual function, reproduction and sexual response. These are the androgens (the best known being testosterone), oestrogens and progestogens. Some oestrogen comes from the breakdown of androgens.

Androgen in women comes half from the ovaries and half from the adrenal cortex. It encourages female body hair growth and sebaceous gland activity. It probably encourages the growth of the external genitalia at puberty, including the labia and the clitoris. Small, medically administered doses of testosterone are known to increase the size and sensitivity of the clitoris so it is reasonable to suspect it may also be responsible for sensual feeling elsewhere such as all over the body.

Oestrogen is produced mainly by the ovaries but some is also produced by the adrenal cortex. It is an important source of oestrogens after the menopause when the ovaries have stopped producing it. Oestrogens are responsible during puberty for developing the breasts, and also encourage the development of internal organs such as the Fallopian tubes, the uterus and the vagina. Oestrogen is responsible for producing the vaginal lubrication during the early part of the sexual cycle. Oestrogens probably also influence the growth of body hair, encourage healthy growth of the uterine lining and indirectly trigger ovulation.

78

Progesterone is the most important progestogen and is produced mainly by the corpus luteum of the ovary and by the placenta. Progestogens act alongside oestrogen to promote breast gland growth and subsequent milk production. In the second half of the menstrual cycle progesterone acts on the lining of the womb to prepare it for the arrival of a fertilized egg.

Both testosterone and oestradiol (one of the oestrogens) are affected by something called *sex-hormone binding globulin* which literally binds these two hormones rendering them mostly inoperative and leaving only very small amounts of each hormone to be free-ranging and therefore to exert their influence on our bodies. This is the normal state of affairs but rarely, due to an inbalance of sex-hormone binding globulin, too much of the testosterone and oestradiol is bound which means we may lose sexual desire or find that our physical sexual characteristics are immature. Medical intervention can re-balance the system in some cases where this happens.

Hormone activity at each life-stage

Hormone activity during childhood

During the early years levels of sex hormones remain low for both sexes. It is only as children mature that sex hormone levels rise, as they do at puberty.

Hormone activity during puberty

Girls growth spurt at puberty occurs roughly two years earlier than that of boys. It also ends two years earlier. In practical terms this means that because girls start the growth spurt from a smaller height they end up, on average, as shorter adults by comparison. The heightened amounts of oestrogen that circulate in girls between the ages of 9 to 13 years are linked with breast development while the onset of the ovulatory cycle begins between $11\frac{1}{2}$ to $15\frac{1}{2}$ years. The general fluctuations of hormones settle into a regular pattern at the time of the onset of periods but has been shown to do so before actual menstruation begins—in a type of practice run for several cycles.

Hormone activity during adulthood

The pattern of hormone activity during the menstrual cycles normally remains consistent until the menopause, barring events such as pregnancy, breastfeeding or going on the pill. (See chart on page 82 for details.) Each month the proportions of the three main hormones rise and fall at the same intervals of time unless something goes wrong so, for example, there is always a peak of oestrogen shortly before ovulation and testosterone is always high in the last two weeks of a menstrual month.

Hormone activity during menopause

The average age for the onset of menopause is around fifty but with a wide variation (between forty and sixty years). The actual changes in the cycle are generally believed to begin not earlier than forty and to finish not later than 60 but there is new thought which argues that these hormonal changes may be more gradual than previously suspected. One factor leading to this theory is the observed increase in strength of the changes in body and mood which regularly occur during each menstrual cycle as the years progress. What may only have been faintly noticeable at twenty becomes an established menstrual pattern by forty.

The common pattern of menopause is for the menstrual flow to become less until it finally stops. Some women may also have 'periods' less regularly before they stop completely. The ovaries stop producing oestradiol although they continue to produce androgens, which together with other androgens constantly secreted by the adrenal cortex, are converted into oestrogen. Although the overall body levels of oestrogen drop after the menopause there are still therefore large amounts within the body which only decline with time. A study of women who have gone through the menopause found that forty per cent still retained moderate amounts of oestrogen within their vaginas until well into their seventies. Levels of progesterone in post-menopausal women drop to negligible amounts and remain at a low, roughly corresponding to the progesterone level of the first half of the former menstrual cycle.

The effect of hormones on sexual libido

Early childhood and puberty

Tiny *children* are noted to get pleasurable feelings from handling their genitals. Five and six year olds begin to exchange 'lavatory talk' amongst themselves and often get into experimentative sex play around these ages. Since hormone levels remain much the same during this period these developments probably represent a growth in consciousness of sexual feeling already present.

At *puberty* sexual sensation becomes far more intense and although deliberate masturbation among girls may be delayed because of learned inhibition, unconscious masturbation (in bed with a doll or with a hot water bottle) may develop.

Influence of the balance of hormones

One argument says that women who have extra androgen within their bodies are likely to possess the strongest sex drive while those with little androgen are likely to have a much weaker sex drive. How our 'allotted amount' is decided is a matter of speculation but influential factors suggested are inheritance, hormonal environment during conception and pregnancy, and the effect of early conditioning on the brain.

Dr John Bancroft of Edinburgh University has observed that men possessing less testosterone also possess less ability to fantasize erotically and Dr Alan Riley, editor of the *British Journal of Sexual Medicine* speculates that women who enjoy giving their partners fellatio may actually become more highly sexed since the semen they take in orally contains testosterone.

It is also theorized that progesterone may lower our libido and, although small amounts of oestrogen may be necessary for retaining normal libido, fluctuations in oestrogen levels don't appear to affect libido in the adult woman.

Changes during menstrual cycle

The menstrual cycle itself, a carefully balanced fluctuation of the three sex hormones plus a variety of others (mainly at and around ovulation) indicate that high spots of the menstrual month for sexual interest are immediately before the onset of a period, around and during the period and for the first half of the cycle. Some women experience another burst of interest during ovulation but studies show a decline in sexual interest during the last half of the menstrual month when progesterone levels are increasing. The accompanying chart shows how the three hormones rise and fall during a menstrual month.

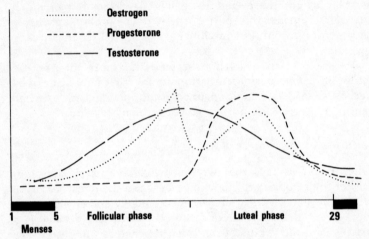

Normal pattern of hormone changes during the menstrual cycle.

Changes during pregnancy

Changes in desire during *pregnancy* are described in Chapter 7 while libido changes during lactation are probably influenced by the post-birth scarcity of oestrogen, and perhaps by the effect of another hormone, prolactin.

Changes caused by the pill

There is convincing argument that the pill, although the *easiest* choice of first contraceptive for young women, is also feeding their hormonal systems with extra hormone at a time when their bodies are trying to establish their own regular monthly pattern of hormonal function. On the other hand, babies born to early teenage mothers can also cause long-term problems so the choice is a difficult one. Introducing young men and women to barrier methods of birth control in a sensitive manner in early teenage might prove a healthier alternative.

Much debate exists at present concerning the effect of the pill on sexuality. Some pill users say that their sexuality has improved as a result of knowing they are unlikely to conceive while others perceive a lessening of sexual interest as use of the pill persists. One study of pill-users showed that thirty per cent of the women taking part became depressed while on the pill. Depression in turn depresses sex drive and inhibits sexual response.

There are also strong links between pill-taking and thrush. Constant painful thrush disrupts sexual relationships and in extreme cases, prevents sex altogether.

Dr Ellen Grant, formerly of the Neurology Department of Charing Cross Hospital, has stated that the pill seems to produce severe migraine and multiple food allergies and that this effect might be related to alterations in the liver function.

Changes caused by ageing

After the menopause, ageing does affect female sexual response but the degree of change varies with each individual. In most women, there is less vaginal lubrication as a result of lessened oestrogen and this can lead to painful intercourse (see Chapter 4). This dryness of the vagina can be treated with oestrogen creams (locally applied) or with HRT (hormone replacement therapy). Both treatments efficiently restore lubrication so that intercourse becomes pleasurable again. Various studies have found that sexual interest decreases with age, with working-class women tending to lose interest faster than those in other classes. A Danish study found that marriages where sexual activity had declined, were invariably influenced by the wife's loss of interest. Whether or not this gradual decline in sexual interest is the result of dwindling hormone levels has not been ascertained. Masters and Johnson have stated that the sexuality of older women is positively or negatively affected by a variety of circumstantial factors and the existence of numbers of older women with continuing sexual interest would seem to bear this out. HRT incidentally, while it does restore oestrogen levels and vaginal lubrication, does *not* restore sexual interest. However, if androgens are the hormones mainly responsible for sex drive it could be that replacement testosterone might facilitate pleasurable sexual response. Clinical experience shows this to be the case.

Hormone related problems

Dysmenorrhoea (period pains)

Many women suffer from mild, cramp-like period pains at the base of the spine coupled with a draining, sinking sensation. But a few young women experience extreme dysmenorrhoea while the cramping spasms seem to fill the abdomen and the sufferer has to lie down in a curled-up position until the spasm relaxes. The pain may persist for only a short time or, more often, necessitate the young woman taking a half day or even a whole day off school or work. The experience is debilitating and even frightening.

Usually these extreme period pains wear off during the teenage years and by the twenties the sufferer is free of them. But there are cases of unpleasant period pain persisting until the age of thirty.

The pains are due to a release of natural prostaglandin for the expulsion of the menstrual blood, and in these difficult cases the sufferer appears to be producing more prostaglandin than is strictly necessary.

Secondary dysmenorrhoea, also a form of abdominal pain, is associated with a variety of gynaecological conditions such as endometriosis (painful abdominal condition where fragments of the womb lining attach themselves to other parts of the pelvic anatomy), pelvic inflammatory disease or fibroids (tumours consisting of fibrous and muscular tissue). Women with extreme abdominal pain should always seek early medical examination.

Treatment Aspirins and other anti-inflammatory drugs (frequently used to treat arthritic conditions) have recently been found to possess a mild antiprostaglandin activity and are therefore the best type of painkiller with which to quieten period pains. Sufferers from constant pain, however, should beware of overdosing on aspirin.

PMT (Premenstrual Tension)

Many books have been written about Premenstrual Tension (PMT) (some of which are listed in Appendix 2). There is still a great deal of controversy concerning PMT and 'cures' are constantly being 'discovered'.

The most up to date explanation of PMT is that it is a collection of syndromes under the umbrella name of PMT.

Symptoms Symptoms are usually felt for seven to ten days before the beginning of menstruation and sometimes continue for a couple of days after bleeding has begun. There are also some women who feel the same symptoms but in the middle of their cycle (at ovulation time) which then usually clear up although, in certain cases, they persist without a break until menstruation commences.

The symptoms can be physical, mental or both. Some women may have many, others just one or two. Most women are mild sufferers and can manage without any help or dose themselves with Vitamin B6 which has been shown to help certain types of PMT. A very few women have extreme PMT symptoms bordering on a type of madness.

Estimates which state that eighty per cent of all women have PMT at some time or other in their lives and that PMT is an illness, should be disregarded. Since women are subject to regular hormonal cycles it is probably normal that moods and physiological changes should occur in moderation. Also, these *are* only estimates—no true census of women's menstrual health has ever been carried out. Finally, the implication that all PMT is an illness is positively harmful. PMT is only an illness where it seriously impairs health and lifestyle. And this occurs only in a minority of women. The symptoms of PMT can include the following:
- Fluid retention
- Breast swelling and tenderness
- Swelling of hands and feet
- Persistent headache
- Skin problems
- Loss of co-ordination
- Depression

85

- Food cravings
- Irritability
- Aggression
- Tension
- Easy crying
- Compulsive behaviour
- Difficulty in thinking
- Forgetfulness
- Clumsiness.

There are many others and one US study suggests there are at least forty-seven symptoms.

In 1983, American researchers indicated that there are probably four main subgroups of PMT. Professor Guy Abrahams, a former US professor of obstetrics and gynaecological endocrinology, listed these as:

- PMT-A: characterized by anxiety, irritability and tension;
- PMT-H: weight gain, abdominal bloating and mastalgia
- PMT-C: increased appetite, fatigue, palpitations and headache
- PMT-D: depression, withdrawal and suicidal inclinations.

PMT-A is associated with high levels of oestrogen and low progesterone. Professor Abrahams observes that administration of Vitamin B6 at doses of 200–800 mg a day reduce the oestrogen level, increase progesterone and resulted in improved symptoms. Women in this group consume a great deal of dairy products and refined sugar. Cutting these out is advised and he suggests progesterone may also be helpful to them, used alongside oestrogen.

PMT-H, characterized by fluid retention, is associated with high levels of serum aldosterone, a hormone secreted by the adrenal glands. Vitamin B6 at a high dosage suppresses aldosterone and prevents the retention of fluid in the tissues. Salt and sugar should also be avoided; salt because it increases fluid retention and sugar because it intensifies the fluid-retaining activities of the salt. Drugs which block the effect of aldosterone may be helpful e.g. spironolactone.

PMT-C, characterized by food cravings, over-eating sweet substances followed by headaches, fatigue and sometimes palpitations or the shakes, is associated with increased carbohydrate tolerance and a low level of magnesium. Magnesium supplements improve sugar tolerance and decrease PMT symptoms and help eliminate the food cravings. PMT-C may also be associated with a deficiency of the prostaglandin PGE1. Cutting out animal fats and increasing the consumption of vegetable oils increases cis-linolenic acid (a nutrient important for the production of PGE1) within our systems. Oil of evening primrose is also beneficial.

PMT-D is the least common but most potentially at risk group, characterized by depression, insomnia, forgetfulness. In one study it was associated with low oestrogen levels and high progesterone levels. In addition, progesterone levels were higher than normal in the middle of the cycle. High levels of adrenal androgen were observed in some PMT-D patients who also had problems of hirsutism (excess hair). Two PMT-D patients of Professor Abrahams also had high lead levels in their tissue and chronic lead intoxication although their hormone levels were normal. Professor Abrahams suggests careful and individual therapy for each PMT-D patient, among these are possible oestrogen supplements. In cases where lead was a factor he argues that it is plausible that a deficiency in magnesium could predispose someone to chronic lead intoxication because magnesium blocks lead absorption.

PMT and sexual desire A common experience of many women is that their sexual desire (libido) dwindles towards the end of their menstrual month and is regained once the period commences. Whether or not this is a part of the premenstrual syndrome is uncertain. However, the Pre-Menstrual Tension Advisory Service noted that loss of libido was reported so often by the women writing in for advice that they decided to make a study of this particular aspect of the menstrual month.

They selected fifty women who had reported loss of libido among a host of other severe problems. The women received appropriate nutritional advice and were surveyed at the end of a three month period:
- Half of the women reported complete return of their libido.
- A further nineteen (thirty-eight per cent) reported a significant improvement.
- Six reported little or no improvement.
- No one experienced any further deterioration.

This was not a controlled study and it is therefore possible to argue that any improvement is due to the placebo effect and may not last. Nevertheless, the improvement was there and one woman even reported being reunited with her husband from whom she had separated shortly before going on the diet because of her pre-menstrual problems.

Whether there is more PMT about these days than formerly cannot be determined. Many more cases seem to be reported and speculation about the causes range from the pill to the stress involved in living in a competitive world. (Regular constant exercise such as jogging goes a long way to reduce stress levels.)

Treatments

Progesterone. Dr Katharina Dalton, the UK pioneer of PMT therapy, has claimed excellent results using progesterone treatment with patients suffering from extreme PMT. Other studies, however, have shown progesterone to have little effect and a recent double-blind trial failed to establish progesterone as having any better effect than a placebo. Some women claim progesterone increases rather than decreases their symptoms.

Oestrogen. Mr John Studd, consultant gynaecologist at King's College Hospital, London, using oestradiol implants (organon) on women with the type of PMT characterized by menstrual migraine, tension and depression found that eighty-four per cent of the subjects reported complete or almost complete relief from their symptoms. Mr Studd believes that sudden lack of oestrogen may be responsible for post-natal depression also and has stated publicly that he is of the opinion progesterone actually makes women with PMT feel worse rather than better.

Vitamin B6. Controlled trials have shown that Vitamin B6 is effective at improving PMT symptoms in many users and, as Professor Abrahams has made clear, it seems specially effective with PMT-A and PMT-H, the two most common subgroups.

Evening Primrose Oil (efamol). It was discovered by accident that doses of gamma-linolenic acid (an essential fatty acid) greatly helped certain PMT sufferers. At present, it is only found in evening primrose oil. Trials are being carried out at present to ascertain its worth. In a preliminary study carried out at St

Thomas's Hospital PMT clinic sixty per cent of women reported excellent responses and a further twenty per cent a useful partial response.

Danazol. This drug is a purely synthetic steroid which completely suppresses the menstrual cycle. It is not suitable for widespread use but is very helpful for extreme cases.

Diuretics. Water eliminating drugs are often suggested in an attempt to prevent the bloating which is such a common symptom of PMT. However, although they do enable the sufferer to excrete water more efficiently they do not appear to alleviate any other of the symptoms.

Nutrition Therapy. Professor Abrahams' nutritional approach to PMT involves classifying what kind of PMT subgroup you fall in to and then, following the subsequent nutritional approach. For details concerning this see the previous pages.

Keeping a menstruation diary for a couple of months and noting down the specific symptoms is helpful in categorizing your subgroup. Specialist advice about this approach can be obtained from the Pre-Menstrual Tension Advisory Service who are at present the only British organisation specializing in Professor Abrahams methods of treatment. (See Appendix Two for address.)

General self-help. Smoking and excess caffeine intake may be implicated with severe PMT symptoms. So, too, may lack of exercise. Cutting out the former, taking up the latter and following a diet rich in fresh vegetables will make you feel generally better even if it does not work miracles for your menstruation.

Post-natal depression

Post-natal depression is usually regarded as a psychiatric problem. One theory says it is the result of birth being over-'technicalized' and therefore removed from the mother's control. This, the argument goes, throws her into a depression. But Mr John Studd, of Kings College Hospital, London, believes that the sudden absence of the hormones oestrogen and progesterone immediately after the birth may be responsible for triggering off a depression. He points out that in his study group of women being treated for premenstrual tension the incidence of post-natal depression was forty-one per cent, which is four times the accepted rate of ten per cent.

Another theory is that if certain women are receiving too much of a particular hormone then its sudden withdrawal at times ordained by nature may cause withdrawal symptoms and that post-natal depression is an example of this.

There is no evidence to show that women suffer from loss of libido during post-natal depression but that is because no one has ever thought of asking them. Since depressed people are known to lose desire, it almost certainly happens to post-natally depressed mothers. And as with any other loss of libido through depression, the depression needs to be treated before sexual feeling can return. How this treatment is handled is up to the individual sufferer and her doctor.

Treatment In view of the new understanding concerning the role of oestrogen and progesterone it is obviously worth considering hormone therapy.

The menopause

Although there is a gradual decline of sexual interest and ability in later years it is not as abrupt as used to be thought and many marriages function on a sexual level very happily for many years after the menopause. Women with these continuing sexual marriages do appear to have two things in common:

● They have a partner who is actively interested in having sex with them
● They enjoyed good sex lives *before* the onset of the menopause.

However for some women the menopause does make sexual relations temporarily less easy. It is estimated that about eighty-five per cent of women suffer one or two of the classic symptoms of the menopause. These are usually experienced between the ages of forty-five and fifty-five, the average age being about forty-nine. The climacteric—the period of hormone transition—usually lasts for about two-and-a-half years but for some women the symptoms last for as long as five. The actual cause of the climacteric (change of life) is the gradual and natural withdrawal of oestrogen from the body due to the ovaries ceasing to function as hormone manufacturers.

Symptoms These may include hot flushes and excess sweating, headaches, loss of memory and concentration, vaginal atrophy (the vagina dries and shrinks), anxiety, loss of sex drive, depression, insomnia and bladder disturbances.

Most of these interrupt a sex life but some more so than others. Vaginal atrophy is the direct result of the withdrawal of oestrogen from the tissues and can result in painful intercourse. Women who enjoy regular intercourse do not seem to become dry as quickly as those who are less sexually active. Loss of sex drive may result from the menopausal drop in testosterone levels. Work by John Studd of King's College Hospital indicates this *is* the case.

Another finding by Mr Studd, in his surveys of menopausal women, has been that women approaching the menopause attend the clinic with many more *psychological* complaints than women who have already gone through the menopause and generally have *physical* complaints.

Self-help treatments Readers not wishing to use hormone replacement but preferring to rely upon more old fashioned remedies might note that Vitamin E was once the menopausal treatment of choice. Although there has been no research which confirms this some women claim Vitamin E taken regularly prevents hot flushes. A suggested dose is between 30 to 100 mg. On no account should more than 100 mg be taken, however.

Claims for other hormones, in particular B6, are also made to alleviate menopausal symptoms but present nutritional trends argue that a carefully balanced diet that includes necessary vitamins, proteins and calcium is better than taking vitamins etc. in pill form. Be that as it may, it is possible to take B6 and calcium supplements. B6 pills tend to vary between 50 and 100 mg in dosage and only a low dosage should be necessary. Some experts believe that B6 dosage needs to be adjusted gradually, starting with a low dosage but making it higher if the low amounts don't have much effect. The dosage should not, however, go above 200 mg and many people think it shouldn't be more than 100 mg. Calcium, too, can be taken as a supplement if you don't think you get 600 mg of it from daily cheese, milk and butter. Working out a daily eating programme that isn't going to encourage you to put on quantities of excess weight but is going to provide you with necessary protein, vitamins, minerals and folate may well balance the worst excesses of the menopause and for specific suggestions of how to do this, see *Menopause* by Raewyn Mackenzie (Sheldon Press).

Recognizing signs of stress which are exaggerated by the menopause is useful. If you can alleviate the stress, then you feel much better about yourself as a maturing woman. Exercise is one way of getting rid of stress, talking emotional problems through another. In New Zealand there is a movement to form self-help groups for menopausal women because the shared experience of talking things through, making friends and feeling supported has proved to be so beneficial to the participants. We could do worse than follow their example. Assertiveness training is helpful, and so too are regular relaxation exercises—while getting a sensible amount of rest is vital at this stage of life.

HRT (Hormone replacement therapy) Hormone replacement therapy, consisting of oestrogen combined with some progesterone taken orally, has been successful for years now in relieving the main menopausal problems such as vaginal atrophy, hot flushes, depression. Local applications of oestrogen cream to the vaginal tissue can also restore elasticity, thus allowing intercourse to become comfortable and pleasurable again. What has not always been restored by either of these treatments is libido.

Recent work by Mr John Studd and associates has shown however that oestradiol and testosterone implants do two jobs:
- Release needed extra oestrogen (oestradiol) in a slow and consistent manner over a period of months, thus restoring general health. (The oestrogen is absorbed better by this method than when taken orally, when it is often poorly absorbed into the bloodstream.)
- Release testosterone (which has little effect when taken by mouth) which restores libido completely in two-thirds of all patients complaining of loss of desire. In addition, oestradiol appears to eliminate headaches in women who suffer meno-pausal migraine.

Women with oestradiol implants who have not had hysterectomy also have to take progestogen for seven days each month to safeguard the lining of the womb. The only side effect of the whole treatment—an increase in body hair—came from the testosterone and the dosage in Mr Studd's tests was altered to take this into account. The increase in body hair was 'no more than a slight increase in downy facial hair' and 'was always improved when the dose of testosterone was halved or discontinued in subsequent implants'.

Double-blind trials to prove the superiority of oestradiol and testosterone replacement over placebo established without doubt that it was the hormones which allowed these menopausal women to feel better rather than any *belief* that they were receiving treatment.

Hormone replacement has also been shown to prevent the loss of calcium that causes bone deterioration in mid-life and later. It also protects the skin in old age, allowing it to retain the elasticity of youth and to protect against heart attack.

Cancer fears In the early days of HRT when women were treated with oestrogen alone there were dangers that they might develop cancer of the womb. However, as soon as this was understood, progesterone—which allows the womb to shed its lining in a monthly bleed just as it does during a normal period—was added to the therapy. Subsequent research has shown that some women receiving this combined hormone therapy are actually safeguarded by the additional progesterone since it can be shown statistically they would have developed cancer of the womb. HRT has been shown to offer protection also against heart disease. The only indication that HRT is not suitable would be if there is any likelihood of thrombosis or some breast cancers.

Menopause clinics

For a list of menopause clinics see Appendix 2.

New hormonal research

Testosterone

The activity of testosterone in both sexes, says Dr Alan Riley, is regulated by a substance called hormone binding-globulin, which binds the majority of our testosterone making it sexually ineffectual. The small amount left becomes free-ranging (sexually) throughout our bodies and is responsible for our sex drive.

Since our hormones are finely balanced by each other, a slight malfunction in one of several hormones can be responsible for greater amounts of binding-globulin in the bloodstream to need 'feeding'. This extra, binding globulin seizes upon some of the free-ranging testosterone and binds that, too. The result is very little is left over to give us our usual feelings of sexuality.

The solution is to re-balance the system by giving a calculated amount of testosterone, but this is not easy to achieve. Although, as John Studd has demonstrated, hormone implants are an effective way of conveying small amounts of testosterone to the bloodstream, it is difficult to determine how much extra testosterone is needed. Since every woman is an individual there is no hard and fast rule about how much she requires and the dose is usually arrived at by trial and error with a high degree of clinical judgement by the doctor.

Another method once experimented with in Australia was intended to help women regain sensuality in their genitals. A testosterone cream was recommended to be rubbed on to the clitoris. The results were spectacular. Sensitivity increased most successfully and the women thus treated were able to experience responsiveness and easy orgasm without difficulty. But ... they also developed facial hair and deepening voices. The hormone therapy had to be called to a halt, since it became apparent that this method of application fed dangerously large doses of the hormone into the bloodstream.

Most research on the effects of testosterone on women has been done while using testosterone alone. But testosterone is metabolized by oestrogen and it is possible that effective testosterone therapy needs to take this into account. In Australia an Australian GP and sex therapist, Dr H. R. Bailey, has used an androgen-oestrogen combined preparation on women who were unable to respond sexually. By using this in combination with psycho-therapy, sex education and anti-depressants where appropriate, he is obtaining an eighty per cent success rate. Usually, just three or four doses of the hormone preparation are sufficient.

UK studies have shown that testosterone tablets dissolved under the tongue, have shown very poor results probably because the dose has been too low, and this may strengthen the likelihood that implants or intramuscular injection are the only reliable methods of introducing testosterone efficiently into the body.

Research that has measured the amounts of testosterone before and after ovulation and before and after menstruation show that sexual activity peaked before and after menstruation but that this was not necessarily dependent on testosterone levels.

Prolactin As mentioned in Chapter 7 (Pregnancy) high levels of the hormone prolactin may be responsible for diminishing sex drive. Pregnancy is not always responsible for creating this condition and, if there is a cause for concern, prolactin levels should be examined during blood sampling. Treatment for conditions other than pregnancy with the drug bromocryptine usually lowers the prolactin level, and sometimes results in a dramatic improvement in sex drive and response.

Blood tests to establish hormone levels

In order to get an accurate assessment of how women's hormone levels are balanced, very careful blood tests need to be taken. Since hormone levels fluctuate at different times of the month it is important to take this into account. In addition, hormone levels fluctuate not just with the time of the month but also with stress. One of the causes of stress is having a needle pushed into one of your veins in order to take a blood sample!

Alan Riley suggests the following procedure should be adopted.

1 The needle should be inserted but then left in place for several minutes without drawing blood so that the client can get used to the experience and relax.

2 Using this method, blood should be taken on not one but on at least three occasions during the menstrual month.

3 The blood from all three occasions should then be pooled for analysis. (It is not possible, he states, to get an accurate assessment with only one blood sample.)

Theories of inheritance

It may sound strange to theorize that sexual libido could be inherited but anthropologists are arguing that this may be so. If it were possible to establish that individual bio-chemistry *can* be passed on through the generations, then it is plausible to deduce that libido is inherited since it is beginning to look as though libido is developed as the result of certain hormone combinations.

However, since it is impossible to know whether or not grandmother suffered from an over-abundance of sexual desire, there is not a lot of use to be made of such a theory. In addition, stress has been shown to affect hormone levels and modern civilized life is agreed to provoke far higher stress levels than existed in previous centuries. Furthermore, there is an interplay between our spontaneous level of sex drive generated by hormones and psychological influences caused by social mores and upbringing, etc.

Advances in oral contraception

The effect of Vitamin C Vitamin junkies who believe in self-dosing with large amounts of Vitamin C should take note of a new finding that large doses of C can convert a low-dose oral contraceptive into a high-dose one. While remaining efficient as a contraceptive, the pill now becomes a health risk.

Oral contraception for epileptic women has been a problem because the anticonvulsant drugs they also have to take may provoke break-through bleeding and thus contraceptive failure. One way of getting over this problem is to prescribe a high dosage oral contraceptive (possibly a 50 mg preparation) for two cycles. If breakthrough bleeding still occurs, this can be increased to 80 mg or even 100 mg a day. This, states Dr Michael Orme of Liverpool University, is quite safe. Because of the enhanced metabolism of epileptic women, it is *not* like giving a high dose to non-epileptic women.

The effect of antibiotics on oral contraception is a problematical one. About forty pregnancies have been reported in women on antibiotics. But so far, no research has illustrated how the antibiotics cause this reaction. Pill-users are warned to use some other contraceptive method as well as the pill if they have to go on to antibiotics and, for safety's sake, for a further two weeks after the end of the antibiotic course.

A new progestogen called desogestrel has been used in the contraceptive pill called Marvelon (30 mg oestrogen plus 150 mg desogestrel). This has proved very useful for women with problems of hirsutism. It is well-tolerated, decreases superfluous hair growth and does not promote hair growth in normal women.

Breast cancer and the pill Swedish research shows that there is a significant increase in the incidence of breast cancer among women who started to take the combined Pill at an early age. Their data suggests the risks increase eleven-fold in women under twenty when they start the pill but gives firmer evidence of a three-fold increase in women starting at twenty to twenty-four years of age. The study also showed that women starting the pill after a first pregnancy had a *lower* relative risk of breast cancer.

English research now suggests a possible doubling of the risk of *cervical cancer* in women who took the pill for more than eight years. These most recent studies though have been criticized by Dr Malcolm Pike of the Imperial Cancer Research Fund who says that not all factors with relevance to sexual behaviour were taken into account when assessing the women studied and that the incidence of factors such as genital warts among the partners of these women, was not assessed at all. Genital warts, stated Dr Pike, are the most likely cause of triggering cervical cancer. He also adds that regular breast checks and cervical smears are able to ascertain the likelihood of cancer rapidly enough to catch it before it becomes serious.

SEVEN

Pregnancy and Sexual Response

Physiological changes during pregnancy

During pregnancy, alongside the rapidly developing baby, go other more subtle forms of expansion in the body. Separate physiological changes occur at varying stages.

The earliest changes affect the *breasts*. In the first three months they increase in size by 25 per cent due to tissue and glandular alteration. So, too, do the nipples. In women who have not previously given birth this breast enlargement can be a painful experience and the breasts feel sore or tender. The tenderness decreases, however, during mild and late pregnancy. By the time the pregnancy is nearly over, the breasts will have increased by almost one-third of their pre-pregnant size.

In a study of six pregnant women by Masters and Johnson, all six reported highly increased levels of sexual tension in and around the *genitals* from the fourth month onwards. The researchers deduced from this that the process involved in supporting the weight of the child creates unusually high levels of sexual tension.

By the end of the sixth month all six women reported strong sex drives, resulting in a variety of orgasmic experiences. Their genitals had increased in size due to sexual congestion and all reported greater vaginal secretion. The researchers thought this latter development to be due to the constant state of sexual arousal in the lower pelvis.

Their findings also show that women between the fourth and ninth month of pregnancy experience far higher levels of sexual tension than non-pregnant women. This may mean that those of us who normally find it hard to experience orgasm, may be able to do so with ease during pregnancy. It may also mean that some women will experience multiple orgasm for the first time. However, because the vagina is so constantly swollen, it cannot contract very forcefully which means the climax itself may not feel particularly intense. In contrast, contractions may be sensed with unprecedented strength in the uterus.

During the last three months of pregnancy, especially during the final weeks, the *uterus* (womb) may move differently during climax. Instead of contracting regularly and rhythmically as it does on most other occasions, it may go into a long spasm. It may remain clenched in a particular position for as long as a minute. Therefore, orgasm may prepare the uterus for child-birth in that it provides a rehearsal of long-held contractions during labour.

Whereas the bodies of non-pregnant women return to their normal, uncongested, relaxed state, after climax, the bodies of the pregnant women in the Masters and Johnson study did not. Despite orgasm, the sexual congestion in the pelvis and genitals was often not totally cleared. The more advanced the preg-nancy was, the less the congestion cleared. This accounts for the almost continual feeling of restlessness that some women acquire towards the end of pregnancy in spite of enjoying a good sex life.

Hormonal changes during pregnancy

There are massive hormonal changes in pregnancy. The placenta for example produces, in particular, oestriol (the oestrogen of pregnancy) and quantities of progesterone. Progesterone reduces the excitability (reaction to stimulus) of the lining of the womb and probably, therefore, plays an important part in maintaining the pregnancy.

Oestrogen and progesterone together stimulate the growth of the breasts and uterus of the pregnant woman, and oestrogens probably stimulate blood flow through the uterus. The levels of free-ranging testosterone in the body fall slightly. One school of thought is that our levels of free-ranging testosterone are responsible for sex drive. If it *is*, this would mean pregnant women are likely to experience decreased levels of sexual interest and response. Numbers of studies, other than those by Masters and Johnson, demonstrate a gradual decline in sexual interest during pregnancy.

Sex problems during pregnancy

There are many additional factors that influence the pregnant woman's interest in sex. One study showed that women who had never previously experienced pregnancy were the most likely to lose sexual interest. One reason for this could be because most women continue to go out to work during a first pregnancy and the stress that both the travelling and the occupation itself produces, can create a reservoir of *fatigue*. Indeed fatigue must be the major reason why pregnant women—despite all the additional sexual tension described by Masters and Johnson—don't become over-interested in sex. It is perfectly possible to have great physical need for sex but to be so exhausted that the sex act becomes impossible.

Sore and tender breasts Particularly during the first three months, this problem can make foreplay and intercourse painful experiences. When you consider that in addition to the pregnant state of being 25 per cent sexually tense (by non-pregnant standards), there is also full sexual tension on the breasts, the total stress adds up to 125 per cent—and a very uncomfortable female. For couples who have set up a sex pattern which includes a lot of playful 'grabbing' and 'handling' this can prove difficult. Explain this to your husband and remind him if necessary, reassuring him it is not so much *you* who needs to play things down temporarily but your bosom. It should help you both, to understand that this is a temporary occurrence, that the extreme tenderness will diminish and that the breasts do eventually return to normal.

Overall fitness prior to pregnancy also affects the mother-to-be's sense of well-being. If you are exercised and strong, and eating a light but nourishing diet, you stand a far better chance of enjoying sex than if you are overweight, lacking in exercise, eating heavy, unsuitable foods and are smoking. No pregnant woman or, indeed, a woman planning pregnancy, should smoke anyway. Smoking has harmful effects on the foetus.

Some women are unwilling to acknowledge that pregnancy in any way changes anything and struggle on through every pre-pregnant activity however unsuitable or uncomfortable. It is not so much actual fatigue that this produces as feelings of stress. Stress can affect sexual desire.

Some men feel that the baby comes between them and their partner (as it does literally) when lovemaking. The fact that during the latter stages of pregnancy intercourse is only possible in a complicated 'scissors' position or with a rear entry position can also deter your partner.

Uncomfortable physical state
As pregnancy progresses many women begin to grow very uncomfortable with their physical state:
● Their backs may ache.
● Their feet swell and hurt.
● Their legs feel as if they are no longer capable of supporting a big belly.
● Rest may be difficult to obtain because of the difficulty in finding a comfortable resting position and because of movement by the baby itself.

None of these encourage feelings of sexual desire. But they are *temporary* conditions.

Safety of sex during pregnancy Some women become extremely protective of the child they carry within them and see intercourse during pregnancy as an invasion that will threaten the unborn. Some men, too, fear that the thrust of intercourse may actually harm the child and you should both be reassured that this simply is not the case. There is no scientific evidence that orgasm can cause miscarriage although there are theories that climax can prepare the uterus for birth by strengthening muscular response. Unless you are otherwise counselled by your doctor there should be no reason why intercourse cannot be continued up until a month before the birth, and the same is true of masturbation. Some doctors are now uncertain about the desirability of sexual intercourse during the last month of pregnancy since there may be some connection between this and babies born with certain respiratory disease. This link has not been proved, but it does seem sensible to play safe.

If there is any bleeding during intercourse the doctor should be notified immediately. He will probably advise you to discontinue intercourse until the pregnancy settles down again and may advocate bed rest. Women with a history of miscarriage are often advised by their doctor to refrain from intercourse in the first few months of pregnancy.

Post pregnancy effects on sexual response

Physiological changes

The following, temporary bodily changes are common. Simply knowing in advance that they are likely to occur, can be a great reassurance.

The breasts After childbirth, the woman who does not breastfeed and who suppresses her milk artificially takes far longer to respond with normal sexual tension in the breasts than does a breastfeeding woman. Some women find that during sexual excitement at this time, their breasts respond by involuntarily spurting milk. This is a normal response and indicates that your body's 'sexual system' is in good working order. Non-breast-feeders don't experience such a strong breast response until months later.

The genitals lose their high degree of sexual tension and their sexual response is slower and longer. There is a reduced quantity of vaginal lubrication, less alteration in shape of the vagina, and erection and tension of the labia and clitoris may be delayed until the plateau phase (shortly before orgasm), instead of developing much earlier. This means that despite feeling sexual desire it becomes harder to attain orgasm. Nevertheless, sexual response and orgasm are still possible if you have a sensitive partner.

Studies show that between the 10th and 12th week after pregnancy, the normal sexual response returns, although it always returns more slowly if you are a nursing mother. Despite the slow re-awakening of sexual feeling breastfeeding women report, nevertheless there is a high sexual interest and emotional desire.

Hormonal changes

Suckling is a sensual activity that stimulates production of the hormone oxytocin, which in turn releases milk. Oxytocin is also responsible for producing contractions of the uterus and therefore it is possible that suckling induces changes in sexual response. This seems further likely if one considers the reflex of involuntary spurts of milk from the breasts during excitement —when the oxytocin reflex presumably works in reverse.

The hormone prolactin, which encourages the production of milk, also remains at a high level when you are breastfeeding although the levels drop within three weeks if you are not. When the levels go down, ovulation usually begins a short time afterwards. If you breastfeed this happens on average around the 10th to 12th week after pregnancy. It is also at this time that a heightened (normal) sexual response returns and it is very likely that the two occurrences are related.

One of the reasons that prolactin levels tail off at this time may be that solids are usually introduced to a baby's diet at about the third month and that milk feeds, particularly during the night, tail off in frequency. It may be frequency which is the key to the return of sexual feeling. Certainly African women who frequently suckle their children for a three year period are able to delay conception for that period of time but, as yet, no research has been carried out to investigate if sexual response is also simultaneously delayed.

Sex problems and solutions

Tiredness Having a baby is energy-sapping. It can take anything up to a year for you to regain your former energy levels although this of course depends on many factors: how long the broken nights continue, how much stress you are coping with, how much support you receive within the home, to name but a few. Although it is perfectly possible for you to enjoy sex and have a strong sexual response even when you are exhausted, the likelihood of being able to arouse enthusiasm is distinctly lower than before pregnancy.

The best form of self-help for tiredness is to be prepared for it in advance. It helps to understand that the three months after the birth need to be regarded as the same kind of emergency state as were the last couple of months before the birth. However much you may want to be a cosy family unit, when you discover how tiring it is looking after a tiny baby you will wish you had arranged outside help. If Mother, or friends, or hired help are available, this can make all the difference between coping and collapse. If you have the sort of partner who is capable of taking over the housework on a regular basis during those months—and sharing it thereafter—that, of course, is the best of all. But the 'New Man' still has a long way to go and if yours is positively not a 'New Man' make sure that you do get that help from elsewhere. Do not try to soldier on!

If someone else can do the housework, shopping *and* food preparation in the early weeks so much the better. Having a sleep in the afternoon whenever possible is a wise move. Dropping your standards about house cleanliness is another. Allowing your husband to fully share in the baby care (if he is a New Man) helps. If you are bottle feeding your baby let your partner take over that task too, occasionally so that not every night is a broken one.

Even if you *are* too exhausted for sex it is important for you, as a nursing mother, to emphasize constantly that you love your partner. It also helps if both partners get it clear this is only a phase and one which doesn't last for ever. There is a very good case for occasionally parking baby with granny on a Saturday afternoon and using the time for lovemaking.

Episiotomy Poor suturing after episiotomy (a cut made in the vaginal wall and underlying tissue to avoid tearing the vagina as the baby's head comes through) can create a ridge of scar tissue within the vagina that remains tender for months after the event. This can make intercourse painful and thus diminish sexual desire. (See Chapter 9.)

Regular massage of the affected area with a vegetable based massage oil during the months after the delivery may soften the tissue and help make it more supple. In extreme cases further surgery may be called for, so do consult your doctor if the problem persists. (See Chapter 10.)

Lack of support Young mothers who lack practical support in the home often feel they lack emotional support too. If the person on whom this lack is focused is their partner, the marital situation can become tense and full of resentment. This may lessen the desire for sex.

Setting up practical support systems, in advance of bringing home the baby, helps you to get off to a relaxed start. Avoid letting yourself become isolated by ensuring that a friend or relative calls in each day for the first weeks of the post-natal period. Any woman who can cultivate a group of friends in a similar situation may find that sharing child-care is of enormous value.

Practical support in the home (see under *Tiredness*) also amounts to emotional support. The young father who really helps at home is likely to gain considerably more gratification both sexually and emotionally than the father who retreats, leaving everything up to his wife. A partner's behaviour in the early months can have long-term repercussions on the sub-sequent quality of married life. However, young mothers can also gain a sense of support from other young mothers and feelings of happiness gained outside the home can counteract potential problems within the home. Where two partners are unable to resolve sexual difficulties, however, it is sensible to ask for outside help, as soon as the young mother has recovered from the birth and stopped breastfeeding.

Side-effects of breastfeeding. You may possess a lot of desire but find, as a result of continued breastfeeding (see former section on hormonal changes), that your sexual response is diminished. Since this makes it harder to experience arousal and orgasm it may create problems between you and your partner. The man who is used to his wife's enthusiastic orgasmic response may read preoccupation with the baby as the cause of her lessened response and may react with jealousy.

The appearance of the breasts during lactation, particularly in the early stages, may also deter some couples. It can be hard to see breasts as the sex objects they previously were when they are now being used as objects of utility. This erotic alteration is also reflected in a more general manner when some couples find it hard to distinguish 'mother' from 'lover'. Some men read 'mother' as their own mother and are filled with incestuous anxieties over lovemaking with their wives. Some women feel similarly. The involuntary spurt of breast milk during love-making (see previous section) can also make it difficult to maintain desire.

Discussion of the emotional problems which are caused by

breastfeeding can go a long way towards overcoming them:

- If you are feeling uncertain about your appearance re-assurance from your husband helps enormously.
- If your husband feels nervous about lovemaking with a nursing matron, he can be reassured that your altered condition is a temporary one.
- If you are both depressed by the fatigue that overcomes you, the light at the end of the tunnel can be the knowledge that the sleep problem does improve with time.
- Women with anxieties about their new body image may find it invaluable to discuss their anxieties with other women.
- If you both find you are lacking in desire for each other after childbirth and do not understand why, personal counselling might be indicated. American clinical work carried out with couples who lack sexual desire show that the longer the problem is left, the harder it is to improve things. This indicates that post-natal lack of desire is best tackled soon, once your body has been given a reasonable amount of time in which to settle down.

Occasionally the prolactin levels that accompany breast-feeding do not subside when they are supposed to, and one of the side-effects of this is to dampen sexual response. If a high prolactin level is diagnosed there is drug treatment available which brings down the amount of hormone within the body and restores ovulation, desire and response.

Impotence Some men find it very difficult to feel romantic about the birth canal. What was once a vagina with all its sexual connotations has become an exit for baby and all his/her associated birth gore. Beset with anxieties about penetrating such an area, the father may not be able to penetrate at all.

Discussing such anxieties, combined with simple sex therapy exercises usually makes this only a temporary problem for young fathers. If it isn't, there are a number of books which provide self-help sex therapy methods and sex thera-pists may also be consulted. (See both Appendices.)

Self-image. If you have been used to being slim, carefree and independent, you may be shocked to find yourself looking physically different after childbirth in a manner that may not be particularly welcome. It can be hard to adjust to yourself as a slightly plump matron; some women can't believe their husbands will find a matron sexy. In addition, for the first time, as a new mother you may find parallels between yourself and your own mother. Sometimes both partners see themselves differently. Instead of seeing themselves as lovers, as formerly, they begin to consider themselves more stolid and less romantic. They may each become depressed at the thought of being a parent.

Massive reassurance from the partner usually helps a new mother who is feeling uncertain about how she looks and who she has become. Discussion with other women is invaluable and so, too, is the passing of time. Some women take longer than others to return to their former shape, but eating sensibly and doing post-natal exercises will help to speed the process. If both young parents worry about their 'loss of youth', it is important to remember that this depression is probably due to fatigue. Once the nightly routine settles down and something resembling a normal sleep pattern returns, both of you will begin to enjoy life again.

Jealousy It is common for new fathers to feel jealous of the attention directed towards their newborn and for the jealousy to get in the way of a happy love life. But some women also feel jealous of the baby, should the child receive a great deal of affection from its father, when it appears to be affection withdrawn from the marital relationship.

Sometimes there are good reasons to feel jealous. Among these is the reality that you aren't being paid as much attention as you need. Some of us need more than others, thanks to difficult family backgrounds and when a new baby comes along, those who are needy see baby as a rival. Jealousy is best dealt with by expressing it, talking about it and making an attempt to compromise with altered behaviour. The jealous person is wise to work out for himself/herself the cause of the insecurities. Where do they come from? What is the best way of rebalancing the 'internal' you?

If by ending a job or career in order to have baby, you are feeling a sudden loss of identity (and are therefore needy), then taking up something which replenishes your sense of identity will help (even if that something is just a promise to yourself that you *will* return to work eventually).

107

Arranging your life so that your husband has plenty of spare time which he spends with you, so that you can talk about the two of you, helps. If it is he who is jealous, then paying him similar attention, will go far to reassure him. Once the jealous partner gets this reassurance he or she will begin to feel less needy and more loved. Making love follows on directly from this unthawing.

'Slack' vagina. Some women focus on their enlarged vagina as a source of post-natal marriage problems: 'He says he can't feel anything inside me now, I'm so large'. The likelihood of a woman's vagina becoming so large as to prevent the male from feeling any sensation from intercourse is practically nil. Even if it is wider than previously, sexual response causes the vagina to swell and give the impression of becoming smaller. The complaint is far more likely to be used as an excuse rather than be a real cause and it is usually triggered off by *male* anxieties. Rather than face up to internal doubts about the 'new' relationship, some men focus on their partner's vagina. The percentage of cases where the vagina actually does become larger is tiny—and repair surgery can rectify this problem.

Women who voice this complaint of now being 'so big my husband can't feel anything inside me' invariably have nothing wrong with their genitals. If there are any real doubts on this score a visit to the gynaecologist will reassure you. What your husband is actually saying is that he has doubts about the new relationship of being a father. Drawing him out so that he can express these anxieties while simultaneously offering reassurance may go a long way to provoke a positive reaction. If he doesn't respond though, but continues to shy away from sex, then mutual counselling should be sought so that he gets the opportunity to see his sexual relationship in a wider context than just a genital one.

Female sexual anxiety. Women who were previously orgasmic may find it similarly hard to let go now since they may associate the sex act with conception—and ultimately the pain of labour. If it is remembered, pain of childbirth can be responsible for sabotaging sex. Acquiring good birth control is the first step towards self-help. The knowledge that you are reliably pro-tected from further conception is reassuring. Talking through your fears and taking lovemaking in simple, easy stages also helps.

In this country the official time recommended for couples to recommence having sex after birth is around six weeks. But in France the period recommended is three weeks. Perhaps the best criteria is if the lochia (flow of blood from the uterus) has dried up and both partners are ready to resume this important facet of their relationship.

Natually, if there is any unexpected haemorrhaging as a result of sexual activity after the birth, this should be brought to the attention of the doctor immediately. So also should any other anomalies, such as a possible prolapse, or inflammation of the stitching of episiotomy or tear.

Before starting sexual intercourse, however, couples not intending to add to their family immediately should make certain they are adequately protected by birth control.

Abortion

In the days before abortion was legal it was pessimistically predicted that mass termination would have dire psychosexual consequences on women. Since it is probably true to say that women who aborted prior to the 1967 Abortion Reform Act did so in 'back-street' circumstances, there can be little doubt that these were indeed highly stressful experiences with very depressing consequences. But, in the past 15 years, there have been a number of surveys carried out which found that women, although sometimes experiencing immediate post-operative doubts and depression, suffer absolutely no long term ill-effects. In a survey by Greer et al (1976), the proportion of women whose sexual adjustment was rated as satisfactory before the termination was fifty-nine per cent. Three months *after* the operation this proportion had risen to seventy-four per cent and the researchers reported that the 'improvement' was maintained for up to two years after the operation.

A further survey by Ashton (1980), eight weeks after termination, showed that of those in a continuing sexual relationship sixty-one per cent reported no change in the 'quality of their sexual fulfilment', thirty-six per cent said it had improved and 19 per cent that it had deteriorated. Twelve per cent believed that sexual deterioration was due to the abortion.

Dr Colin Brewer's survey in 1978 of women opting for late abortion indicated that these women (who might be expected to find readjustment harder than those getting a termination in the very early weeks) were far less upset than might be anticipated. In general the surveyed women recovered quickly from the operation without serious disruption to their lifestyle.

Abortion is seen by certain feminist psychologists, such as Carol Gilligan, as a major life event. Making the choice between motherhood or termination can force a woman to a radical evaluation of her life and relationships, and can be responsible for a variety of changes in self-esteem. Obviously, feelings of sexuality are heavily implicated here.

How we react to abortion, however, depends greatly on our society's national and cultural attitude towards it. When Yugoslavian psychologist Sofija Trivunac surveyed Yugoslavian women who had had multiple abortions, she found that some felt they had gained in self-esteem. The more terminations they experienced, the sexier they considered themselves to be. Yugoslavia uses abortion as a method of birth control and the attitude towards the operation therefore is that it is a routine matter—just as is a regular check-up at the dentist. Some women have literally dozens of abortions and do not seem disturbed by the fact.

No research appears to be directed towards the hormonal after-effects of abortion. However, since the body has been put into a state of pregnancy it must go through hormonal changes as soon as it stops being pregnant. How this affects the body both physically and mentally seems unclear. Yet when we consider that the IUD (intra-uterine device) is responsible for *regular* abortion these changes become important, since they may mean that IUD users spend as much as fifty per cent of their fertile lives in a state of very early pregnancy. The IUD is responsible for disallowing the newly fertilized egg from attaching to the womb lining. As yet no one has measured the body changes that IUD users experience in the second part of their menstrual month.

Infertility

One in 10 couples are unable to have children. Before they reach this certain knowledge, most of them will have experienced a period of great stress, grief and marital discomfort. Sex problems are some of the causes of infertility. But the condition itself breeds sexual difficulties.

Sex problems as causes of infertility

Sexual ignorance which results in the *non-consummation of a marriage*, is still, in this day and age, one of the causes of infertility. Couples who believe that intercourse should be carried out in orifices other than the vagina sometimes show up at sexual dysfunction clinics. Occasionally a young couple will think they are having sex in the right place but, because the wife has a tough hymen, the penis will in fact be inserted into the back passage, and neither partner knows that this is not the 'usual method'.

Other sex problems such as:
- Vaginismus (see Chapter 5)
- Impotence
- Severe premature ejaculation before entry
- A low frequency of sex
- An over frequency of sex

may all be reasons why a couple does not conceive.

A low frequency of sex may be responsible for impairment of the mobility and longlife of the sperm while a high frequency of sex is sometimes associated with a low sperm count. Readjusting the frequency of intercourse therefore may be one way of making conception easier. Severe sex problems would best benefit from professional advice.

There has been some debate about how necessary orgasm is as a means of aiding fertilization. There is evidence that as the woman becomes sexually aroused, the PH levels in the vagina change, becoming more receptive to sperm. Sperm survival is helped by this changed environment, although orgasm is not essential.

Other problems as causes of infertility Stress has also been indicated as one of the culprits of infertility but sometimes it can be hard to

111

say which came first, the lack of conception or the feelings of tension. However, research shows that stressed couples who received sex counselling, subsequently enjoyed between forty-five and fifty per cent success in starting a family. Knowing that you have *got* to have sex at a certain time is a pressure in itself and if this is the case, using some of those self-pleasuring techniques which form a basis for other types of sex therapy, may go a long way to bring some of the pleasure back into the act. Group counselling, too, has shown good results for couples suffering from stress and self-help fertility groups might go a long way towards helping would-be parents help themselves.

Then there are the gynaecological problems. Failure to ovulate is one and this can in many cases be assisted with drug treatment. Problems with the uterus or the Fallopian tubes are others. Sometimes these can be helped with surgery, sometimes they can't. Occasionally the woman's cervical mucus turns out to be hostile to the partner's sperm and manages to kill it off before giving it a chance to reach the egg. Specialist advice here may help to change the mucus and self-help theories centre on alkaline douches or even placing a diaphragm containing the husband's ejaculate over the cervix, thus giving the sperm an aided start. If the cervical mucus has actually produced antibodies to the sperm, there are a number of options open. Apart from medically assisted ones, self-help may necessitate the couple using sheaths or condoms for a year in order to allow the mucus to lose its antibodies and become normal before trying again.

In the male the sperm itself may be non-existent, or unhealthy, or there may be a physical blockage which prevents the sperms from release. An excellent book on the subject which goes into all the causes of infertility very thoroughly is Dr Andrew Stanway's *Why Us?* (Granada).

Infertility as a cause of sex problems

Depression plays a part in inhibiting a couple's desire for sex, and depression often hits both man and wife during the struggle to have a baby. Men may feel fatherhood is necessary as confirmation that they are indeed masculine and conversely women may see maternity as femininity at its most extreme.

The dawning realization they may not possess these imaginary sexual qualities as previously assumed can be very depressing to cope with.

'Performance pressure' is an early sex problem to show up when a couple know they need to have sex at a particular time of the month (around ovulation). Sex becomes a chore, losing spontaneity and women react with loss of desire while men occasionally find they are impotent. Frequent gynaecological examinations can make the whole business of trying for a baby seem fearful, and if there were any marital or sexual difficulties previously these can become overwhelming now.

Help for sex problems

If the sex problems aren't discussed at the infertility clinic (which most of them are) they should be specifically voiced. Talking things through with the doctor or being referred on to a counsellor is one way of coming to terms with the emotional difficulties raised by trying for a baby over a long period of time. Voicing anxieties with each other or with outside friends may also be a help. The National Association for the Childless (see Appendix on p. 180) has local contacts who attempt to assist people undergoing infertility treatment. See Appendix on p. 180 for recommended reading.

AID (Artificial Insemination Donor) If AID is acceptable to both partners it may be able to produce a child when all else has failed. This may have the long-term effect of calming down tense couples and allowing their sex life to return to a normal routine. It may alternatively, however, raise questions in the man about the male role and be responsible for extending his sense of marital tension.

Childlessness

The result of understanding you are never going to become parents may either be the break-up of a marriage or a greatly strengthened relationship. In the latter case there is substantial evidence to show that childless couples are physically and psychologically as well off, in some cases even better off, than

113

are their counterparts with children. The National Association for the Childless once again proves invaluable for helping infertile couples come to terms with childlessness over the long term.

EIGHT

The Effects of Drugs on Sexuality

Since mediaeval times necromancers and alchemists have sought for the perfect aphrodisiac—that mystical substance reputed to enhance sexual sensation—and discovered, some say, in the phallic-shaped mandrake root and in a tiger's testicles!

Present-day researchers are, however, still looking. So far, it seems that if a certain drug does seem to aid the libido, it probably does so only in the mind. What the medical profession now understands about present-day drugs is that they may act on our sexuality in one of two ways:

• They may either diminish or enhance the sex *urge*.
• They may impair the *mechanism* that controls erection and ejaculation in men and genital responses in women.

Anti-depressive drugs are good examples of substances which manage to do both. Many patients suffering from depression find that their mental and physical problems are greatly relieved as a result of drug action. As the depression lifts, sexual desire returns. However, in some cases, although the patients now want sex, when they try to have it all may not be in working order. The arousal mechanisms may find it a struggle to provide any real sensation. It is often only when the patient comes off the drug that the ability to enjoy sex and have a climax returns. The anti-depressant restored desire but also subdued response.

Alcohol Perhaps this is the main substance that people think of as an aphrodisiac. It is, in fact, the opposite. Because it is a brain depressant, it acts on the libido in separate stages:

• The first stage, when you've drunk a small amount, removes anxiety from the brain centres, thus removing feelings of worry and inhibition. This may allow sexy feelings to emerge that otherwise would not be given the chance.
• However, with larger doses, alcohol rapidly depresses our behaviour, including our sexual response. This is why, when

115

we retire to bed, after a celebration, we may find we are unable to celebrate any further.

American research has shown that in men, regular excessive amounts of alcohol tend to lower testosterone levels, thus impairing the ability to get an erection. There is no parallel research on women but since women also possess amounts of testosterone and since sexologists now theorize that these may be responsible for part of their sex drive, a similar 'turning off' sex may be experienced by female alcoholics. The alcoholic or even the partial alcoholic (this includes social drinkers) will need to reduce her drinking substantially if she wants to see a satisfactory restoration of sexual sensation.

Barbiturates and other hypnotic drugs have similar effects. In small doses they release inhibitions. In larger amounts, they depress *all* behaviour.

The 'popular' drugs (such as *LSD* and *marijuana*) are often described as aphrodisiacs. So far, most research on this has been conflicting. Certainly, some marijuana users report that 'pot' combines the actions of lowering inhibitions while heightening sexual stimulation.

LSD produces dramatic alterations in the consciousness and perceptions can be intensely erotic, but this seems to depend very much on the stimuli surrounding the 'tripper' and the frame of mind you start off with. Orgasm on LSD tends to be less absorbing and yet a more prolonged and encompassing experience. If the 'tripper' is not with someone she finds erotic and trustworthy, sex experienced on a 'bad trip' can be so terrifying that all interest in sex will rapidly diminish.

MDA, one of the hallucinogens which is amphetamine-related, has been reported to have sexually stimulating effects, but again, it is experienced as part of the whole changed drug experience, not in sexual isolation.

Cocaine sniffing in the US. This is presently fashionable and part of its attraction is that, used sparingly, it can have an unrivalled effect on sexual desire and drive. However, it is easy to become addicted to cocaine and one's entire behaviour state can rapidly change from normality to psychosis. This includes illness, depression and loss of interest in everything including sex. The drug is also corrosive to nostrils and gums.

Bromocryptine acts on the (hormone) prolactin levels of both men and women. By lowering these it can aid impaired libido, infertility problems and obesity.

Spanish fly or Cantharides is a poisonous substance which acts by irritating the bladder and urethra. It is highly dangerous and has caused both impotence and death.

Amyl nitrite (fashionable among society and homosexual circles) is a drug used normally for angina sufferers. Studies have shown that this increases sexual feeling in the genitals if inhaled shortly before orgasm. The same studies also seem to indicate that it is not addictive nor does it do the user any long-term damage, or indeed any short term damage provided they are healthy. However, users with weak hearts who abuse the drug have been known to die of heart attacks.

Many of the drugs used in the prevention and cure of illness impair sexuality and performance as a side-effect. An over-stimulated patient, whose mood has been calmed by *Lithium* may also experience a lessening of sex urge. *Melleril*, an anti-psychotic and anti-anxiety preparation can result in a dry male orgasm. Anti-depressant drugs are also sometimes responsible for lowering the libido. For further details of the chemical reactions that drugs in everyday medical usage may have upon our love lives, see the Drugs Table on p. 118.

While some drugs may not possess unpleasant side-effects when taken on their own, the side-effects become marked if they are combined with alcohol. In addition *many drugs react with each other* so it is vital to check all drug usage with a GP before adding something new. Contraception may be affected by drug usage—most notably strong antibiotics sometimes upset IUD action and certain drugs such as corticosteroids, some anti-biotics and phenobarbitone combined with contraceptive hormone (the pill) produce adverse results.

All in all, there is not a really satisfactory drug which can be safely used as an aphrodisiac without side-effects of any kind. There are, on the other hand, any number of drugs which should be avoided, if you want to maintain a normal sexual response. As sex therapist Helen Singer Kaplan puts it in her book *The New Sex Therapy*, 'no chemical substance has yet been discovered which can rival the aphrodisiac power of being in love'.

DRUGS TABLE

The sexual side-effects of drugs on *men* are also itemized in the following table since, in many cases, the side-effects clearly show up on men but not on women. This is not necessarily because women don't have the same drug reactions but rather that women's sexual response is harder to measure than that of men. We thus have less monitored work carried out in connection with women's drug responses. It is reasonable to assume, however, that if a drug has a particular side-effect on a man, there will be an equivalent side-effect on a woman.

Drug	Effect on Sexual Response
Alcohol	By reducing anxiety small amounts may help sexual response and the ability to climax. Large amounts, however, depress sexual appetite. Chronic male drinkers will become completely impotent and possibly a parallel response happens in women.
Anti-depressants 1 MAO inhibitors e.g. pargyline phenelzine (nardil) nialimide (niamid)	Inability to achieve erection (men) and a lessening of sexual interest (women) may affect a small percentage. Pargyline may delay or retard ejaculation (men) while phenelzine has been shown to increase sperm production in men with abnormally low sperm counts.
2 Tricyclics e.g. clomipramine (anafranil)	Sexual appetite increases as depression lifts, but roughly 20 per cent (men) are unable to achieve erection while corresponding lessening of sexual ability is possible for women.
Antihistamines 1 H1-receptor antagonist (travel sickness remedies) e.g. diphenhydramine (benadryl)	Libido may be reduced and vaginal lubrication impaired.

118

Drug	Effect on Sexual Response
2 H2-receptor antagonist (ulcer healing preparations) e.g. cimetidine (tagamet)	Libido may be reduced and a small percentage of men will be unable to achieve erection.
Antihypertensives methyldopa (aldomet, dopamet)	It is common to lose interest in sex as the dose increases. With a high dosage men may experience problems with erection and ejaculation, while women may become less responsive and unable to have an orgasm.
propranolol (inderal, propranolol hydrochloride)	A small percentage of people will experience lessened sexual appetite (men and women) and inability to achieve erection (men)
hydralazine, (apresoline, hydralazine hydrochloride) prazosin, (hypovase hydrochloride)	Some reduction in libido and some erectile problems (men)
Anti-Parkinsonian drugs levodopa (berkdopa, brocadopa, aradopa, L-dopa)	Libido may increase
Cannabis	Used in small quantities it may increase libido. Reports conflict regarding constant use of large quantities. Some indicate that sexual appetite remains high, others indicate such severe disorientation that appetite is non-existent.
Clofibrate (atromid-S)	Occasionally libido is reduced and difficulties experienced with erection (men)
Diuretics 1 thiazides e.g. bendrofluazide (aprinox, berkozide, neo-naclex, bendroflumethiazide)	Erection (men) and vaginal lubrication (women) may be impaired in a small percentage
2 loop diuretics e.g. frusemide (lasix, furosemide)	

Drug	Effect on Sexual Response
3 spironolactone (aldactone)	With increased doses libido wanes and erection (men) and vaginal lubrication (women) diminishes
Hormones 1 oral contraceptives	Conflicting reports. Some women experience increased sexual desire, others a reduced libido.
2 androgens e.g. testosterone preparations	May restore sex drive and ability to climax in men and women
3 oestrogens	May increase or restore vaginal lubrication in post-menopausal women. May seriously impair male libido, erection and ejaculation
4 anti-androgens	Reduces male sexual appetite and commonly prevents erection and ejaculation
Opiates—painkillers e.g. heroin, methadone	Short term use is likely to lessen libido. Addiction may lead to impotence and sterility. Libido, sexual ability usually returns on withdrawal from the drugs.
Tranquillizers 1 minor tranquillizers e.g. diazepam (valium), chlordiazepoxide (librium), lorazepam (ativan) potassium clorazepate (tranxene)	Effects on libido and performance are slight but variable. Tranxene may be effective in improving diminished libido.
2 major tranquillizers e.g. chlorpromazine (largactil), benperidol (anquil)	Reduced libido commonly occurs especially with benperidol. Delayed or absent ejaculation (men) commonly occurs and high dosage may be connected with inability to achieve erection (men).
Sleeping preparations 1 barbiturates e.g. butobarbitone (sonergan, soneryl, butamet)	Medium doses taken as prescribed over the short term do not adversely affect sexual response Long term addiction however causes chronic deterioration of sexual ability leading to impotence in some cases (men) and loss of libido (women)
2 non-barbiturates e.g. nitrazepam (mogadon)	Generally without serious sexual side-effects

NINE

Illness and Sexuality

Only recently has it been fully appreciated that disease and abnormal physical conditions of the body can produce a deterioration in sexual response. Sometimes the deterioration is a direct response to the physical condition; sometimes it is a psychosomatic response in that some ill people *expect* sex to be diminished.

Recent estimates of people visiting their doctor with sex problems puts the incidence of organic or physical causes as high as thirty per cent. On this basis, anyone suspecting they may have a sex problem would be wise to ask for a thorough physical check-up before going on to seek counselling advice.

The following illnesses are all known to affect sexuality in some patients.

Angina

Angina, where bouts of energetic movement may cause attacks of painful spasm around the heart, understandably restricts enthusiasm about sexual intercourse. Less strenuous sexual activity is one way of dealing with the problem and inhaling long-acting nitroglycerines prior to intercourse may not only reduce attacks but actually enhance orgasm. US research has shown no undesirable side effects when these drugs are taken in moderation.

Arthritis

Arthritic pain sometimes inhibits overall enjoyment of love-making but very often it adversely affects the actual movement of the sufferer, making it difficult for example to enjoy straight-forward missionary position intercourse. Arthritic hips are especially troublesome for women.

The disability can be eased by use of specially prescribed drugs and by having a hot bath prior to lovemaking. Lovemaking can be encouraged to take forms other than intercourse and if intercourse is specially desired then working out which positions are most comfortable and using cushions or pillows as supports is most helpful. Arthritis symptoms vary in intensity during the day and couples are therefore advised to make the most of the least painful periods.

Asthma

Asthma, induced by exercise, may inhibit sexual activity. But in most cases preparation by thorough use of a bronchodilator beforehand, should inhibit an attack and allow relaxed enjoyment of intercourse.

Blood disorders affecting the genitals

Just as male sexual activity is facilitated by a healthy blood supply to the penis, thus ensuring erection when sexually aroused, female sexual activity is similarly facilitated. In order to respond sexually, increased blood flow to the genitals assures vaginal lubrication, swelling of the labia and vaginal wall and clitoral erection.

Although research with regards to blood supply to the female genitalia is virtually non-existent, it is reasonable to assume that just as obstructions to the blood supply of this area affect male erection, they are equally likely to inhibit female sexual response. Arterial disease might be responsible for such obstruction, and so might scar tissue as a result of accidental wounding, or surgery. Third degree tears during childbirth and subsequent repair, general vaginal repair surgery and surgery affecting the rectum may all inhibit perineal blood supply in some way with the side-effect of lessening female response. (See also Chapter 4.)

Chronic renal failure

Uraemia results in a loss of sexual appetite and a general feeling of uncertainty regarding sex activity. Many women develop a degree of sexual unresponsiveness too. Haemodialysis or renal transplant usually restores interest in sexual activity but does not always restore response.

Other treatments such as the use of clomiphene citrate, bromocriptine or zinc may help certain sufferers, but the results indicated so far are usually poor. However, sufferers from renal disease often become depressed as a result of the illness, and in these cases, careful counselling can sometimes lift the depression and aid subsequent lovemaking.

Diabetes

Recent studies of the orgasmic response of women with well controlled diabetes show that there is relative freedom from sexual problems. There is also some indication that diabetic women have more positive attitudes to their husbands than do normal women and that this produces beneficial effects on the sexual relationship, which counteract any stresses also suffered.

However, diabetic women are specially prone to vaginal infections such as thrush which may make intercourse uncomfortable and they also tend to have more hazardous pregnancies and larger than average babies. The psychological effects of these problems on attitudes to sexuality may mean that post-birth sexuality becomes problematical too. In addition, the use of hormone based contraceptives disturbs diabetic control, so that other means such as barrier methods are preferable.

Epilepsy

The majority of women suffering from epilepsy have perfectly normal sex lives and it is very rare for a fit to be triggered off by intercourse or orgasm. However, epileptic sedation can sometimes produce complications and so can difficulties in adjusting to the epileptic state. Fear of orgasm is a usual inhibition in such women. Those who experienced the onset of epilepsy during childhood are more likely to make negative associations between epilepsy and sexuality. This may be due to the more sheltered and fearful upbringing they will have received from parents made anxious by their condition.

Temporal lobe epilepsy however has a definite association with a low or non-existent interest in sexual activity, lack of sexual curiosity, sexual fantasy or sensual activity. Much more rarely, hypersexuality (excessive display of sexual activity) is shown and this sometimes takes the form of an abnormal sexual preference such as transsexualism, excessive masturbation and aimless attempts at intercourse. Women also show difficulty in responding to sexual stimulation. Drug treatment complicates the picture since it has recently been recognized that anticonvulsants such as phenobarbitone affect certain hormone levels and diminish sex-drive.

Heart attack, heart disease

The majority of people with heart disease are capable of enjoying a normal and full sex life. However, a few (who have suffered from heart attacks) may change their attitudes regarding sexual intercourse, through fear that something so energetic will put them at risk of a further attack.

Research shows that sexual intercourse is the equivalent to other forms of moderate exercise. The increase in blood pressure and heart rate around the time of orgasm was actually less than that which occurs during moderate physical exercise. In addition men who went through a physical 'shaping up' programme for overall health, after heart attack, showed a decline in their peak heart rate during intercourse, compared with similar men who did *not* go through such a training. There is no reason to think the condition would differ for women.

There are some grounds for thought that sexual intercourse in stressed situations is more likely to lead to heart attack than regular sexual intercourse with a constant partner. Japanese research shows that, although rare, sudden death during sex, is more likely to occur in an extra-marital sexual encounter when, presumably, stress is heightened.

The psychological effects of heart attack may have an impact on general feelings of well-being. Often the patient, recovering from a first attack, understands that, for safety's sake, an entire way of life needs to be altered. This can be unnerving and disorientating. Combined with feelings of vulnerability and anxiety, these make poor conditions for enjoying energetic activity.

There are rarely reasons why women with heart conditions should abstain from sexual activity provided they are able to improve their overall health. If however intercourse becomes anxiety-provoking, learning to value other less energetic forms of sexual activity, such as mutual masturbation, individual masturbation and oral sex, may be beneficial substitutes.

Hypertension

One of the side-effects of heart disease can be hypertension. The effects of hypertension on sexuality are uncertain. However, some drugs used in the treatment of hypertension appear to interfere with sexual function and, if this is the case, it is wise to consult your doctor and attempt to alter the drug regimen. The woman with acute hypertension may also worry that sexual activity will put up her blood pressure to a dangerous level. In such cases other forms of lovemaking are advisable.

Resumption of sexual activity is best taken in gradual steps. The patient would be wise to begin with solitary masturbation, subsequently practise masturbation with a partner, slowly combining it with gentle intercourse taken at a very easy pace with a lot of mutual caresses.

Multiple sclerosis

About a third of women suffering from multiple sclerosis report difficulty in achieving orgasm, a lowered sexual appetite or reduced genital sensation.

The causes vary from impaired nerve function, to other physical or psychological problems.

As the disorder itself can flare up and die down so, too, can the related sexual disorders. In periods of remission, sufferers should not assume that sexual response is still impaired but should carefully experiment with sexual stimulation. One researcher (Lundberg 1977) made the interesting observation that though MS male sufferers failed to respond to fantasy or erotica with erection, they did respond to genital touch. If a similar reaction is true of women this may mean that some female MS sufferers will not initially feel like sexual activity but if it is nevertheless begun in a tactile manner the response will be there.

So far, treatments of the sexual problem seem to depend on treatment of the problem itself. There have been no sure-fire cures discovered for the condition although, at present, evening primrose oil is enjoying an enthusiastic press.

Spinal cord injury

Spinal injuries appear to affect women sexually less than men. In two major studies, the majority of women reported sexual arousal and lubrication, and a slightly lesser majority in a further study reported very satisfactory sexual relations which included orgasm, although some of them also specified that orgasm had changed in quality since the injuries. The general conclusions from these reports were that many of the affected women, in spite of a difficult period of readjustment, were able to re-establish rewarding sexual relationships. Naturally the mechanics of intercourse are likely to be problematic compared with former activity but sensitive experimentation appears to overcome the difficulties.

Stroke

Strokes are only likely to impair sexual appetite if one small part of the brain is involved. If the stroke involves other areas sexual interest and performance should remain as before. But it doesn't always and anxiety, as a result of the illness, is often responsible for a stressed sexual response. Much of that response rests in the erroneous belief that sexual activity may in some way trigger off another stroke and reassurance that sexual activity is in no way responsible for doing this is often enough to restore a full and healthy sex life.

The sexual side-effects of surgery

Episiotomy and deep tear stitching

The suturing (stitching) after a perineal episiotomy during childbirth or after a tear (as a result of childbirth), can sometimes result in a ridge of hard scar tissue within the vagina. In many cases time will allow this to heal and the over-tender area to settle down. But where it doesn't, there may be an indication for a further minor operation to cut out the excess scar tissue (if this is possible) and to re-stitch it more neatly, so that thick scarring is prevented.

Often, a good time to ask for this repair surgery is prior to the birth of a second or subsequent child when a further episiotomy might be expected. Making certain this request is written in the ante-natal notes should ensure that the operation is carried out. If, however, the scar does not seem so serious, regular massage with a massage oil will help make the area supple.

General surgery

Anaesthesia and the shock of surgery may cause depression. It is common for patients to feel depressed for some months after surgery and depression lowers the capacity for feeling sexual desire and sexual response. Talking through feelings and linking the operation with other life events helps the patient emerge from the depression but in most cases it eventually lifts spontaneously anyway.

Hysterectomy

In most cases hysterectomy (removal of the uterus) improves subsequent sexual experience. The removal of uncomfortable symptoms, fears of pregnancy or uterine disease, results in a physical sense of well-being that extends lovemaking. In a minority though, some sex problems develop. Sometimes these are an extension of sex problems which preceded the operation and some older women regard hysterectomy as a legitimate excuse to 'get out of sex' altogether.

A few women associate sex strongly with procreation (even if, in the past, they have used birth control) and the fact they can no longer give birth may dampen their sexual feeling. Similarly, some women regard the end of menstruation as a sign that they have lost their femininity and do not have the self-esteem necessary to remain a good lover.

Often, post-operative sex problems are the result of mis-information. Careful explanation either from the medical profession or from suitable literature can be of assistance.

Most couples can resume intercourse after six weeks. The vagina may seem narrow and shortened but this is temporary and is resolved with regular and constant intercourse. If intercourse is a problem due to lessened lubrication, an artificial lubricant can be a useful sex aid.

More radical operations such as that which not only removes the uterus but also part of the vagina, may make it harder to resume a sex life. But, providing intercourse is taken slowly and after a greater interval (around three months), regular sex activity will eventually enlarge the vagina to its former size.

Oophorectomy (removal of the uterus, fallopian tubes and the ovaries) has a more extreme sexual effect. Regardless of age, women experience the after-effects as the menopause, and this may be accompanied by a lessening of vaginal lubrication resulting in painful intercourse. Hormone replacement is often one answer to this (and other physical changes) but the use of an oestrogen cream on the vagina can sometimes relieve the dryness problem.

Ileostomy, colostomy, ileal conduit

Occasionally operations may impair sexual response for example if there has been damage due to rectal resection. More often, sex problems are created by the profoundly distasteful situation of having to make love while a piece of tubing which ends in a urine or faeces collection bag is permanently inserted into the abdomen. Women patients are helped overcome their fears and lowered self-esteem if, almost immediately after the operation, their partners can stroke and caress them, making it clear they are still desirable sex partners.

The simple procedure of emptying the appliance before making love can help, as can certain sexual positions. The self-help organization known as The Ileostomy Association, is very supportive to patients with these problems and often instrumental in helping them back to a more positive acceptance of themselves and enjoyment of the sex act.

Mastectomy

Although there is no physical reason why removal of a breast should impair sexual function, it often has far-reaching effects on the female psyche. It is common for women to feel despair on undergoing the operation and a sense of total loss of their femininity. These after-effects can last for years, erode a relationship and sometimes result in total avoidance of any sexual contact.

Although counselling cannot, unfortunately, create miracles, it can help a woman lessen her sorrow and come to terms with her altered body shape. By doing so it may also avert sexual complications. The reaction of the partner is all-important and his involvement with his wife during all post-operative counselling/advice sessions will help him understand what mental pain she is experiencing, help him get over his own feelings and, hopefully, allow him to give continuing demonstrations of affection towards his wife. The couple may be helped if the husband first sees his wife's scar in the presence of the doctor.

Recommencement of sex can begin quite soon, as long as pressure on the wound is avoided. Naturally, positions where the wound/scar is least noticeable, such as the scissors position away from the scar, or the side-to-side position where weight is taken off the wound are desirable.

Radiotherapy

Radiotherapy frequently impairs sexual response since it can result in vaginal fibrosis which prevents the normal vaginal expansion that should occur during sexual response and also prevents vaginal lubrication. As yet, surgeons have no way to overcome this dysfunction.

Rectal resection

Rectal surgery can damage pelvic abdominal nerve fibres. In women, this may produce impaired vaginal lubrication, and occasionally, deep seated pain, owing to lesions affecting the mobility of the upper part of the vagina. There is little so far to help these conditions.

Vaginal repair

Vaginal repair for the treatment of a prolapsed uterus can sometimes result in disturbed sexual activity and response. Sex can become uncomfortable or even impossible if the repair has resulted in a particularly shortened vagina and interior adhesions. However, research shows that women whose surgery is carried out via the vagina rather than via the rectum stand a far greater chance of easy recovery afterwards and an uncomplicated sex life.

Careful post-surgical examination six weeks after the operation should guard against the possibility of interior adhesions and intercourse is recommended at six weeks onwards as a part of the recovery process. Regular intercourse will prevent the vagina from becoming too narrow and will soon allow it to resume its former comfortable shape.

Before going for prolapse surgery, try to ensure that, where it is possible, such an operation is done via the vagina.

Psychological causes of sexual dysfunction

Until recently it was thought that all sexual problems owed their origin to psychological/psychiatric causes. This still appears to be the major reason why people develop difficulties with sexual response although no longer the only one. Chapters 2, 3, 4 and 5 deal with such psychosexual conditions. But there are some mental *illnesses* such as schizophrenia and manic depression, which also have a negative influence on sexuality. These are covered below.

Depression

Depression has an inhibitory effect on sexual behaviour and response. Both appetite and ability to respond may be simultaneously affected although some depressives, while showing little initial interest, discover their response still functions well. Minor depressions are sometimes regularly experienced by women as part of their menstrual cycle and are linked with less sexual desire.

There are many biochemical theories about why depression both in the normal menstrual cycle and in depressive illness is triggered off. And although unproved as yet, there are probably specific hormonal changes, affecting both mood and sexual interest.

However, many people who suffer loss of sexual response through depression may have triggered off the depression in the first place because of an unhappy marriage or unhappy sex life. Either way there is strong cross-fertilization between the two.

Mania is the opposite of depression and manic depressives suffer from both states. Sexual interest and activity is often greatly exaggerated in the manic state and sometimes leads to a loss of inhibition, with displays of inappropriate public sexuality or with a promiscuity formerly out of character. There are a variety of drugs used to control manic depression and psychotherapy, particularly in the manic stage, is valuable.

Eating disorders

Anorexia (where the sufferer may literally starve herself if so allowed) and *bulimia nervosa* (where the sufferer has compulsive binge eating sessions then rids her body of the gorged food either by vomiting or purging) are the two most common eating disorders. Both may be developed by either sex, but both have a tendency to be displayed in very many more young women than men. The origins of these problems are not understood when the problems are self-inflicted.

Both medical research and women's self-help groups, however, have shown an obvious link with sexuality. Body size is linked with sexual attractiveness. Some women find the barrier of their too thin or too large size protects them from subconscious fears of the opposite sex. In the particular society we live in body image has become an obsession and *Cosmopolitan* magazine recently announced it had stopped printing diets on the grounds that the obsession is a dangerous one. The present fad for aerobic sport, however, also feeds the pre-occupation with appearance and it is not unusual to find compulsive dieting linked with compulsive exercise.

Food is also linked with mothering and the theory goes that anorexic young women may be in revolt against turning into a 'mother' like their own. They therefore starve themselves to avoid maturity. However, it is also a fact that by becoming anorexic you place yourself in a kind of 'time-lock'. If starvation continues for long enough you actually revert to 'pre-puberty' since, at a certain stage of weight loss (this varies according to individual body size), periods stop and the body reverts to a childish shape. While this may represent avoidance of identification with Mother, it may also be an avoidance of adult sexual behaviour.

Self-help women's groups have achieved some success with obsessive dieters by enabling the participants to identify for themselves what they are subconsciously trying to achieve with their eating habits.

Some psychiatrists approach the problem of anorexia from a physical (and therefore nourishment) angle and do not carry out any psychotherapy with a patient until she has put back enough weight to re-start ovulation (and therefore her periods). Others scorn this approach as futile and concentrate on what is usually a rich vein of psychological material from the conscious and unconscious. Either way, the condition can be highly dangerous and in extreme cases, fatal. As far as the immediate sexual side-effects of anorexia are concerned, anorexia can be seen as an avoidance of sexuality—indeed a denial of it. There is evidence which shows that women whose weight loss depended on purging and vomiting were more sexually active prior to their weight loss than were those women whose weight loss depended on dieting.

Binge eating is a type of rapid personal gratification and may be a learned way of pleasing or comforting oneself, at a time when there is an unconscious need for gratification. There are similarities here with the habit of smoking and it may be that 'replacement' activities can help some sufferers. (Betty Dodson, the New York sex educator, theorizes that if women substituted masturbation for binge-eating they would be happier and thinner people!) Strategic or intervention therapy has it that by altering the pattern of binge-eating, it is possible to alter the entire attitude of the eater.

Binge-eating and vomiting is seen by psychiatrists as a kind of half-way house between normal eating and anorexia and as such, proves easier to work with.

Little is known about the sexuality of *obese* women except that one study shows obese women were more likely to be sexually assertive. Studies of obese men show, with a few specific exceptions, that sexuality remained average.

Schizophrenia

Schizophrenia itself is not known to cause consistent sexual problems but the drugs used to treat it do. (See Chapter 9 for drug table.) However, the emotional states produced by schizophrenia are so dramatic that individual sufferers are subject to a variety of negative sexual experiences. Someone whose illness has developed in childhood is likely to have less chance of a normal sex life than someone whose schizophrenia develops in later life.

PART 3

*Sexual Role, Sexual Violence
and Bereavement*

TEN

Lesbianism

A lesbian is a woman who loves women and, in most cases, expresses that love through lovemaking. She feels emotionally attached to women, rather than men, and chooses to live with women. Just as a heterosexual may live a celibate life, of course, so too may a lesbian. A lesbian is, in fact, like any other woman except that she prefers women rather than men to be her partners.

Lesbianism in itself is not a problem but because it is not always socially accepted, being lesbian can throw up social difficulties. It isn't easy making the discovery that you love women, breaking the news to parents, friends and relations. Heterosexual adolescents often find it hard to gain confidence and make relationships with members of the opposite sex— even within the context of a society that sees heterosexual mating as desirable. When society is instead deeply suspicious of your preference and likely to be unhappy about it, it is not surprising that your first lesbian relationship is fraught with uncertainty.

Getting started

Some women put off socializing for years, choosing to live lonely and unhappy lives. Others take the risk and tell their friends, hoping they won't be rejected. Many girls find this hard to do while still at school, fearing the reaction of their fellow pupils. They wait until they are older and possibly away from their local group.

Once lesbian feelings are disclosed there are some standard reactions which very young lesbians can expect to hear. One of these is the 'it's only a phase' train of thought. 'You'll grow out of it.' This can be confusing for two reasons:
- It casts doubts on your assessment of your own character. If you can't rely on you, who can you rely on?
- There is, occasionally, a chance that this opinion may prove to be right. Which is doubly confusing.

Even if the latter is true this reaction doesn't help. If, at a later stage you are going to discover love for the opposite sex, you will stumble over it anyway. It is important therefore, to keep a firm grasp on the validity of your own feelings. If, at the age of sixteen, you feel that you are a lesbian, then that is your feeling. Should you wish to change your mind at a later date then you are perfectly entitled to do that, too.

The likelihood is that most women with strong conviction about their sexual identity at such an early age will remain constant with their self-assessment.

Telling your parents

Telling your parents is the next hurdle. How to do this depends on the kind of parents you have. Many people advise breaking the news in a very personal way. Instead of saying bleakly 'I am a lesbian', it may be gentler to say 'I've fallen in love—with a friend who happens to be a woman.'

If you have the kind of parents who you know will cut you off and never speak to you again and if this is going to be unbearable for you, it may not be appropriate to tell them at all. Occasionally, sadly, this happens: one Jewish father for example read 'kaddish' the Jewish prayer for the dead when he learned about his daughter's sexual identity.

But, for all the disowning parents, there are more with positive reactions. A 75-year-old mother ringing in on London Broadcasting's problem phone-in revealed that she suspected her forty-year-old daughter was a lesbian. When asked how she felt about this she said, 'What difference does it make? She's my daughter.' That was one child who might have confided in her parents years ago. Another mother, when told by her 22-year-old daughter, said, 'As a matter of fact, there have been times when I have thought I was too,' and she has been supportive ever since.

Of course, there is an intermediate reaction where parents—particularly of younger teenagers—are deeply unsettled by the news. They may insist on their child seeing a psychiatrist, ground her at home and forbid her to see lesbian friends. They go through awful conflict but do eventually accept, if not endorse, their offspring's personal rights in the matter.

There are various counselling and self-help organizations

138

who help young lesbians over the hurdle of telling their parents. The names and addresses may be found in Appendix 2.

Loneliness

Loneliness is one of the saddest problems to affect isolated young lesbians. Coming out in a small community is often impossible and it is not always possible to move away. Undoubtedly, it helps to live in a large town or city when starting a lesbian lifestyle. This enables women to meet other lesbians, to create a social life and to live exclusively with other women without feeling constantly objects of censure.

The self-help organizations (in particular Lesbian Line) are extremely helpful to lonely women wondering how to go about feeling less alone. Moving to a town is likely to be high on the list of advice, putting yourself in line for parties, clubs, political movements. The principle of this is that through meeting people, you can gain confidence and new friends, as well as avoiding isolation. Living in a town may merely be a stage. There's no law to say that once you are feeling more confident or have found a permanent partner, you shouldn't move back to the country where by now you are likely to be far better mentally equipped to deal with the 'notoriety' of being lesbian.

For those readers who feel strongly that lesbianism shouldn't be a cause for 'notoriety', I am the first to agree. Unfortunately, not everyone else thinks like this yet and still needs to grow comfortable with the idea.

Older lesbians

Not all lesbians discover their sexual identity as teenagers. There is an army of married women whom time and the security of marriage has allowed to discover lesbian feelings of love, when they are nearer thirty rather than twenty. Often such women go into their first lesbian relationship believing themselves to be bisexual. Indeed, many are. But there is also a transition from absolutely straight housewifery through bi-sexuality, sometimes years later, arriving at lesbianism.

Rae Larson, a clergywoman from the West Coast of America, tells of her own 'measuring-stick' for sexual identity. Rae started off dating boys, having long-term relationships and, of course, sex with them. Sex was satisfactory but the feelings behind it never seemed very special. In her twenties Rae decided she was bisexual and developed a close relationship with another woman. This was followed up by another and another. During this time (about eight years) Rae was also having sexual friendships with men.

As the years went by, however, Rae became more and more involved with her women friends and less and less interested in long-term relationships with men. 'Somebody asked me whom I felt the most passion for,' she explains. 'I had had far more sex with men and, on Kinsey's rating, I was a borderline bisexual. But when I considered for whom I had felt the most passion, there was no question about it. It was only ever women. And I realized I wasn't bisexual at all. I just hadn't been able to accept I wasn't part of a heterosexual world. Now there's no problem. I know I am lesbian.'

Bisexuality

Of course, there are many women (and men) who are truly bisexual. They are happy to live with either sex, to have sex with either sex, to feel love for either sex. Being bisexual though undoubtedly complicates relationships. Some people think that bisexuals have an excess of sexual energy—there is so much that some of it spills over to the same sex. Whether or not that is true, many bisexuals have real needs for multiple partners. Perhaps they live with a primary partner but have a variety of other relationships. You need to be a very special spouse indeed to cope with that kind of a lifestyle. The happiest female bisexual I know is married to another bisexual (male). They apparently feel fine about giving each other sexual licence although, as time has gone by, they have lost interest in a very active extrovert sex life and have become much more family orientated—with each other. They still have 'other friends' but the urgency has gone out of extra-marital adventures.

Sex problems

Lesbians, like anyone else, possess their ratio of sex problems and technically these are much the same as those of their heterosexual sisters. But there are some special aspects of lesbian lifestyles which increase certain sexual dilemmas.

Perhaps the most powerful of these is a sense of isolation. Many lesbian women have repressed their sexual feelings for years or have dared to discuss them with only a very few. In these circumstances when one such lesbian meets another, needs for love and touch are released after years of emotional starvation.

Although this may result in the heights of passion, it also often means intense mood swings. Love and hate travel side by side as a result of the real insecurity felt by lesbians who have had to survive in an unfriendly world. This means that lesbian relationships suffer from more than their fair share of jealousy, paranoia and vulnerability. If there is also a ¬ex problem it often gets magnified by these strong feelings.

Most of the sex problems experienced by lesbian women will have already been discussed in this book. (For partner read female partner in the text and ignore the sections referring to sexual intercourse.) But there are some sex problems which crop up often with lesbian women and which are viewed by the women concerned rather differently to those experienced by heterosexual women.

Fear of letting go during lovemaking is one of them. When someone feels very insecure, has perhaps felt 'damaged' by the reaction of others to her lesbianism, it can be hard to trust. The act of opening up to orgasm is a supreme act of trust and not all of us can do that. If the relationship is long term and serious this can get very distressing. Practising mutual pleasuring exercises together, with the emphasis taken off orgasm is helpful (see Appendix 1). So too is careful examination (together) of past events which may link into fears of vulnerability.

A variation of this problem is when the woman is scared about being lesbian and unconsciously interprets orgasm with another woman as some kind of 'final proof'. This fear may provoke enough anxiety to prevent lovemaking from ever having a satisfactory ending. Individual self-pleasuring work helps women gain a different perspective on sexual pleasure (see Appendix 1). Many women who discover their sexual response through their own pleasuring begin to see that the experience of having an orgasm doesn't indicate anything about their nature except that they are fully functioning sexual beings. Sometimes transferring the ability of masturbation to lovemaking continues this new perspective at its most practical level and allows the practitioner to get used to climaxing in the presence of their partner. From there the step to doing this mutually is a small one.

Fear of urination. Since making love with fingers tends to be far more versatile than making love with a penis, one of the problems that sometimes arises with women lovers concerns the G-Spot. In the 'old days' (circa 1975) women used to believe they were urinating during climax and found this very hard to accept. Nowadays it is known that a sensitive area inside the vagina—about two-thirds of the way along the upper wall— yields rapid orgasm in some women if pressed in a certain way. Sometimes it also results in the woman ejaculating a thin arc of pale liquid. This, US experts tell us, is the G-spot response.

Whether it is urination or the G-Spot hardly matters, but some lesbian women have been known to react to this by never allowing their partner to touch them genitally, with the result that they only ever experience climax during private masturbation. Accepting that G-Spot response is a valid form of sexual response is the most straight-forward method of dealing with it. Simply stating to a new partner that you have a G-Spot sexual response and therefore it makes sense to caress and cuddle with towelling between you and the bed is the easiest and the most direct method of getting over this hurdle. If you can accept it, this goes a long way to allowing other people to accept such a response. Incidentally, turning G-Spot exploration into a kind of game for both of you can help take the embarrassment out of the situation. *The G-Spot* by Ladas, Whipple and Perry (Corgi) is full of fascinating information on the subject.

Unrealistic expectations We all possess myths about sexuality. Among the lesbian ones are that there are certain ways in which lesbians ought to make love:
- One woman thought it vital that both partners should climax simultaneously and felt a failure when this turned out to be virtually impossible.
- Another woman with a similar train of thought, believed that lesbians *ought* to make love in the sixty-nine position.

- A common myth is that one partner ought always to take the lead and initiative in loveplay and that the other should allow herself to go where invited to follow.
- Heterosexual sex has brainwashed many women into feeling that some kind of phallic object needs to be included in female lovemaking for the experience to be a 'whole' one.

Common sense makes it clear that as long as sex pleases the two of you, it doesn't matter how you make love, who takes the initiative, whether or not sex aids are included, or if you take turns. One of the lovely aspects of first discovering lesbian lovemaking is that all preconceived ideas of lovemaking can be discarded, conferring the freedom to invent something all of your own.

Lack of fullness Of course, there are some people who feel something *is* missing even when they have enjoyed the most wonderful oral or manual sex. If this is the case, after careful negotiation with your partner, the acquisition of dildo or vibrator may be a helpful purchase. (Mail order addresses for sex aids may be found in Appendix 2, p. 176.)

Dislike of fullness and/or sex aids The opposite problem can occur when one partner prefers using a sex aid and the other doesn't. Negotiation is once again the answer—and compromise. What's good for her needs to be readjusted for you.

Inadequate stimulation Many women believe that stimulation for women needs to be done sensitively and gently. Very often this is true but it isn't the preferred method for *everyone*. Some women like an extremely vigorous-to-the-point-of-being-rough stimulation and therefore what may be right for you may be totally wrong for a new partner. Approaching new sexual relationships with an open mind and exchanging information about how lovemaking feels is the best way of finding out.

Nor does the sex act have to rely on touch stimulation alone. There are stories to tell, jokes to exchange, words of love to express, fantasies to enter into together.

Use of sex aids Mail order catalogues will demonstrate the wide range of sex aids available, but the most effective of all is the vibrator and as long as it is possible to vary the speed almost any kind will do.

Most women use vibrators mainly on the outside of their genitals, gaining maximum stimulation from the effect the vibrations have on the clitoris. Some women use the vibrator inside the vagina while also making love with their hands. Some women like lovemaking face-to-face, body-to-body with genitals rubbing against each other. If this sometimes leaves something to be desired, a two-headed dildo is reported to work wonders.

It is important to keep an open mind where sex aids are concerned. Some women get the impression that sex aids are the invention of men and that their use amounts to making yourself somehow vulnerable to men. Naturally use of sex aids is entirely an individual preference but it may be worth giving them a try.

Emotional problems which affect sex

So many emotional problems affect sex that it is not practicable to catalogue them all. But one of the major emotions to affect lesbian women is that of *jealousy*. Many lesbian women feel insecure when starting to form relationships, as do many heterosexual women. But for the lesbian the 'anxiety stakes' are increased by the ever-present knowledge that her lifestyle is not endorsed by the 'straight' people she is in touch with every day. However strongly you feel about your sexual identity it doesn't stop the early years from being fearful subconsciously.

Even though you have rationalized your behaviour and feel absolutely fine about it, the emotional 'base' from which you work is shakier than that of a heterosexual counterpart. When you feel insecure, you are a prey to jealousy. Jealousy can get in the way of lovemaking, spoil potentially beautiful experiences and make people lose their desire for each other.

When dealing with jealous behaviour it is important to consider not just what are the immediate circumstances that have provoked the outburst, but also that jealousy means a partner is specially needy. Helping a partner to work out personal reasons for this neediness (not just those concerning you) is the most constructive way to deal with jealousy. Be tolerant, patient and encourage the jealous one to build up her self-confidence. Assertion training is helpful here. (See Appendix 2 for addresses.)

Many lesbians have felt very *rejected* by their parents' reactions to their daughter's choice of lifestyle. Sometimes, it is possible by going back for discussion, time and again, to work parents through their initial sad feelings and regain their pride in their daughter. When that happens the daughter starts feeling a lot better in herself too. And a lot less insecure. So if parents' rejection is at the root of your jealous behaviour, it is worth plugging away at their attitudes too. If parents are unable to do this, however, talking through your feelings with friend or counsellor is invaluable.

One of the beauties of a lesbian relationship is that because society expects nothing of you, you and your friend are free to make up the rules for yourself as you go along. Sorting out expectations, agreeing wherever possible on issues like other friendships serve to give each other guidelines about what is expected, even if they aren't adhered to rigidly.

But even partners with the most clearly laid 'regulations' sometimes find that experience alters things. If for example, you resent your friend's behaviour, even though you have no real ground to make an objection, you may be able to learn something about yourself. *Resentment* unfortunately gets in the way of lovemaking. It may be necessary to 're-negotiate' your rules in the light of your strong feelings. Getting a partner to fall in with your new train of thought may not be easy. But then, neither is trying to make love when you are angry and resentful.

Sexual health

Of all women who enjoy an active sex life lesbians are at the least risk of sexually transmitted disease. Apart from the celibate, lesbians are the least likely people to get AIDs, for example. And although diseases such as gonorrhoea can in theory be transferred during oral sex or mutual masturbation it is less likely to occur and indeed, would only occur if the carrier had been particularly promiscuous, or was bisexual.

Naturally, health problems affect everyone and most of Chapters 9 and 10 on illness and drug reactions are relevant to lesbians.

Having a child

Perhaps the area which is most different for lesbian women is that of children. A lesbian lifestyle means that the question of children becomes a big problem area.

One option is to acknowledge that since it is impossible for two women to conceive, childlessness will be part of the chosen lifestyle. But lesbian women often *want* to be mothers and if this becomes important other alternatives have to be considered.

The first question is whether your partner also wants children. If she does, the next question is, how to manage it. Some women simply find a likely man, enter into a brief relationship, and once conception has taken place, just as casually end it. If there are no lingering connections between the two and if he is not named on the baby's birth certificate then the problem of conception has been easily solved.

Unfortunately, life isn't so tidy. People have a way of catching up with you or keeping in touch. Mutual friends, if they know of the connection, may be responsible, even innocently, for letting him know there is a baby on the way. These days men want to be involved with their children and the conceptual father needs either to be a *very* reliable friend or someone from whom all tracks are thoroughly covered.

The objection to this is aesthetic. Not every would-be lesbian mother wants to have sex with a man even in such a good cause. This is where AID (artificial insemination by donor) comes in. Some doctors are willing to help lesbian women become pregnant by this method, but lesbian women themselves are learning to practise AID without the help of a doctor. All that you need are a disposable syringe (available from any surgical supplier) and a willing donor. There is nothing very difficult about douching yourself with ejaculate once these ingredients are present. The risks of this method are that there is still another person involved—the father. Some women cope by employing a go-between, by not divulging their address and by finding the donor through classified advertising. It is difficult territory however and one of the problems which occurs in later life, is how to deal with the child's question: 'Who is my father?'

Lesbian women who consider these options and who reluctantly decide not to follow them up have to face the painful emotional hurdle of childlessness. The National Association for the Childless can help here with sensitive counselling and advice.

For women who do opt to become lesbian mothers there is a Lesbian Mothers group in Manchester (see Appendix 2) and individual women's switchboards may be able to put lesbian mothers in touch with each other. (See Appendix 2.)

Lesbian support

Realizing that all over England, other lesbian women exist who will support and befriend, is the most nurturing information a young lesbian can be given. Getting in touch with others, hearing what happened to them, reading about their lives, gaining inspiration from the way in which other women have dealt with being lesbian in a heterosexual world, are all ways in which you can begin to feel good about yourself. As far as specific sex problems are concerned any lesbian woman can go for sex therapy to any of the sex therapy agencies—in theory sex therapists should be comfortable with all aspects of sexuality and certainly those who are members of the main counselling organizations are.

ELEVEN

Rape, Incest and Exhibitionism

Rape

The victim

Most rape victims are teenage girls or children of either sex, but victims may be of all ages, including women in their 70s and 80s. A high proportion of rapes (around 80 per cent) contain violence. Studies show that violence is more likely if it is a group rape or if the rapist is a stranger. Vaginal intercourse is the most likely act but anal intercourse, forced fellatio and other variations also take place.

There is a variety of opinion about how women should deal with rape while it is happening. One attitude, until recently traditionally displayed by the police, is that women ought to put up the maximum fight possible in order to display unequivocally their resistance to the act. Certainly, screaming or shouting in a public place may scare off the rapist. However many rapes take place in areas which are not public and such resistance may, in these circumstances, serve to anger the rapist who is already violent. Understandably, many women fear doing this since their health and life are in danger.

One of the present anomalies of sexual law in this country is that a wife cannot be raped by her husband in English law, in spite of the fact that rape in marriage is frequently an extension of other marital violence. The best help married women can expect in this situation is to take refuge in a Battered Wives house. There is a pressing need for legal reform.

The rapist

A British study of rapists shows that they are mainly young men. Forty per cent were aged seventeen to twenty and nineteen per cent twenty-one to twenty-four years old. Of these rapists, fifty per cent of them were known to the victim, being either friend, acquaintance or relative. Reasons suggested for their motives vary from a need to feel personally powerful, to aggressive tendencies, traumatic upbringing, sexual irresponsibility, a hatred of women, a specific sexual satisfaction. Studies have not shown any deep-seated pathological reasons for the rapists' actions.

After-effects of rape

Physical Extreme cases may include injuries to the genitals and face and is more common to adult women victims than to children. Permanent physical disability as the result of rape is rare. Alcohol plays a big part in violent rape, the rapist in many cases being heavily under the influence. A few women conceive as the result of rape.

Psychological The immediate effect is trauma and shock. Some women react with far more distress, however, than others. Even if the reaction is rational and controlled, the long-term effects cannot be forgotten. The main subsequent anxieties are an inability to feel safe and extreme anxiety. Some women get extremely depressed, others find it very hard to visit the area where the rape took place, and sexual problems are common. The UK Women's Sexuality Workshop observed that four out of two hundred women attending the workshop had experienced rape, a statistic of one in fifty of women presenting with sexual difficulties. (The sexual problems were those of inability to experience orgasm during sexual intercourse, although the same women were able to climax during masturbation. Two of the four women were strippers, an occupation chosen years after the rape experience.)

The stigma of rape cannot be regarded lightly. Even in this age of concern about rape, plus a more enlightened attitude on the part of the police and networks of rape crisis advice centres, the stigma still holds for many women. The memory of the humiliation experienced may die hard and if repressed may make even more of an impact on the individual. It is best for the victim if the experience can be discussed and feelings brought out into the open.

Rape counselling

Personal counselling, preferably with people experienced in the trauma of rape such as members of a rape crisis centre, is advisable as soon as possible. Rape crisis centres provide the opportunity for one-to-one discussion and for group discussion. In addition, their contacts are available to those who have immediately been through the trauma and also to those who experienced it years previously. (See Appendix 2 for addresses. See also Chapter 3 on Lack of Desire for suggestions for self-help sex therapy with rape victims.)

Social basis of rape

One of the most distressing sides to the phenomenon of rape is that there are many indications that rape is a learned behaviour. Certain tribes are brought up to use sex violently and to rape any woman who is not a member of the tribe. Rape is used as an act of war by soldiers who, under normal conditions back home, wouldn't dream of doing such a thing. The background of war, with its brutality, the realism of killing and being killed all provide the basis for breaking down the usual conventions and allowing other activities to replace them. In other words the conditions of war can amount to brainwashing.

If rape is a learned behaviour then it must follow that demonstrated violence in everyday life can serve to instil and reinforce this learning. Violent pornography therefore, by this deduction, would be part of the educational process.

Two American studies show that sexual offenders (rapists) were sexually aroused by reports of rape or films of rape and that when asked to suppress their sexual response to rape stimuli, they were incapable of doing so, unlike the normal viewers who could. Furthermore, when both groups watched unaggressive stimuli, neither group were particularly moved until they were asked actively to suppress sexual response, at which instant the sexual offenders showed an *increase* in their response. The normal viewers did not.

These findings could indicate not only that rapists are specially aroused by scenes of violence but that the knowledge they shouldn't be, actually increases their response. If this is applied to any man with a tendency to enjoy aggressive sex, it is frightening potentially. Just what makes some men respond to aggressive stimuli in the first place while others do not, is still a mystery. Science fiction suggestions that men ought to be allowed legitimate channels for their violent aggression, such as war, war games or games of violence, bear some consideration. So, too, would the removal of alcohol from all cultures. Violence seems to be largely a constituent of male make-up and is used against women and children who are seen as the weaker components of society. How this violence might be eradicated, while still preserving the human urge to persist and explore, is also science fiction material. Until society becomes female-dominated, however, there is unlikely to be much active research along these lines for obvious reasons.

Incest

Three hundred cases of incest a year are reported for England and Wales, although incest crisis workers believe this represents only a small proportion of the actual cases.

Relationships between brother and sister are probably the most common although these rarely come to court. Mother-son relationships do occur but are rare whereas the majority of reported cases are those between father and daughter. Such a relationship tends to begin when the father is middle-aged and the daughter reaches puberty. In many such cases it does seem that wives unconsciously encourage the situation and notably don't report such activities even though they must know what is going on. Over-crowded conditions appear to encourage incestuous activities and although some incestuous fathers are evidently psychopathic, this is not true of all. Alcoholism plays a part in as many as 50 per cent of such cases.

Short-term consequences

Physical pain, shame, fear, depression, a feeling of being unacceptable to contemporaries, difficulties in making friends (particularly with boys or men) and the likelihood of pregnancy.

Long-term consequences

These are unclear. How a daughter reacts to incest often

depends not so much on the relationship itself as to how it is handled once it becomes public knowledge.

- If the *disclosure* is traumatic, the victim may find it very hard to settle down to a normal life afterwards.
- If the *experiences* are traumatic, however, the victims may have massive incentive to make their own subsequent relationships work well and securely.

The famous story of Noreen Winchester who killed her father for attempting to continue an incestuous relationship after years of incest contrasts with that of another Irish woman personally known. The latter at the age of 11, also experienced an incestuous relationship with her father for two years while he was between wives. Yet she appears to have emerged from this and an otherwise very traumatic childhood relatively unscathed. When asked about the incest she explained that in the part of Ireland where she lived it was unspokenly accepted that incest happened and that it was virtually the eldest daughter's duty to stand in for the mother. Perhaps this local acceptance plus the fact that the incest ended without trauma, helped her to overcome the experiences and dismiss them.

Be that as may, the Incest Survivors Group tells some horrendous tales of entire families of as many as thirteen children, regardless of gender, being sexually assaulted by their father, and it is as a result of this growing consciousness of the problem that a Child Assault Protection programme has been set up (see below).

Sexual consequences

There are no clear statistics setting out an obvious relationship between sex problems and incest. Of four incest survivors personally known, all were able to enjoy a normal sexual response. One is a lesbian, another a croupier/high-class call girl, one a social worker/housewife, the last a professional nanny/housewife. It is worth noting that this gives a ratio of 50 per cent having taken up lifestyles that were sexually 'different'. Such a tiny percentage is, of course, worthless in general terms but a large study on the same lines would be interesting.

Prevention

Since the greater proportion of incest victims are children, the importance of educating them in how to deal with child molesters, be they relations or otherwise, has become urgently apparent.

Clear instruction needs to be given about how not to respond to strangers, how not to accept the invitation of people you know without checking first with mother, how to tell mother of any incident which doesn't feel quite right even if it involves a close relation. For more details of how to do this the Child Assault Prevention Programme has published an excellent booklet *Preventing Child Sexual Assault*. (See Appendix 2 for details.)

Self-help and counselling

Older victims of incest might find it helpful to talk about their past experiences with a close and concerned friend or with other similar victims. Through the Incest Crisis Line and the Incest Survivors Group, the latter is now possible. Concerned mothers, who fear incest is presently taking place in their family can talk through appropriate action with the same groups.

In cases where incest is suspected, it is vital for the child's sake that the activity is stopped and if this means disclosure to someone outside the family (not necessarily the police) this is a small risk to take in order to avoid much greater danger. Often the subject is not brought out into the open within the family because the mother is afraid of both physical violence and the disruption to marriage and family. Since it is understandably difficult to act in these circumstances it is vital that she seeks and gains support before making a move.

But the move needs to be made. In some cases this can be as simple as saying to the incestuous relative 'I know about your activities or intentions and you have got to stop.' If this initiative is ignored, the next step is to say 'If you don't stop what you are doing I will involve the police.' Sadly, if it proves necessary, the final step is to call in the police and social work authorities. On no occasion should you allow a child or teenager to be brutalized sexually by an older or stronger relative.

153

Advice, counselling and befriending can be obtained from Incest Crisis Line and the Incest Survivors Group (see Appendix 2).

Exhibitionism

The traditional view is that most exhibitionists are male and that women exhibitionists are rare, but a more thoughtful view perceives that while the exhibition of women's bodies is socially acceptable that of men's is not. Women *do* dress in front of lighted windows with the curtains open, they *do* sunbathe topless in public places. There is never a problem in finding centrefold models or page three incumbents and there are fashions of 'streaking' in public places.

In general, *no one minds*. Exhibitionistic women don't usually find themselves prosecuted by the police, nor do they cause grievous psychological harm. In fact, some women get *paid* for their exhibitionism. Not all strippers show their body just for money; some do it because they get a sexual kick out of the experience.

Men, on the other hand, are seen to be threatening when they exhibit their private parts. Dominating mothers and subservient fathers are sometimes suggested to be psychological influences on such men while one study observes that boys from orphanages are more likely to 'flash' than other boys. Some men are compulsive flashers, having presumably fixated on their genitals as objects which can shock and control. Others only do so at times when they are suffering an emotional shock. Exhibitionists are described in one study as being immature (in attitude and looks), probably married to a woman who is older, at least in appearance. Inadequate personality is another explanation, although this ignores the fact that some male exhibitionists enjoy happy and normal lifestyles without a hint of inadequacy.

Why exhibit?

An explanation of the tendency in both sexes may hark back to the days of childhood. Part of normal childhood experience is in playing sex games around the ages of five to seven. Showing off genitals is usually part of this and the reactions of other children are included in this play/learning process. When an adult needs to make an impact, perhaps he/she returns to these playground activities. Maybe the active repression of such activities by punishing adults caused such a child to stick at this infantile stage and the knowledge of shock and repression subconsciously makes exposure very attractive.

Therapy

Such behaviour contains an element of challenging the family since the majority of flashers must be aware of the social repercussions if caught. Job, family and friendships are jeopardized and if the would-be flasher is to control such behaviour, analysis is advisable. Certain psycho-sexual units in larger hospitals specialize in counselling exhibitionists and referral can be made to them by the GP. In some places self-referral is possible.

Self-help

Most exhibitionists are locked-in to their behaviour, finding it impossible to confide. Yet talking about feelings, the need to be loved, perhaps a former problem of neglect by partner or earlier still by mother, is all fruitful. Learning to feel better about yourself by feeling accepted by your confidant helps prevent such extreme displays.

So, too, does firm and explicit detail of the legal and social consequences of such acts. The majority of exhibitionists taken to court, don't appear there again. They have presumably learned the hard way to control themselves. Perhaps spelling it out in advance therefore would have a preventative effect.

The problem with self-help is that the exhibitionist has to own up before any of this can be put into practice. It may not, alas, be possible to practise prevention before there is already some social scandal.

Victim

The vast majority of male exhibitionists are harmless; exposure of the sexual parts being an end in itself. While these experiences may be momentarily shocking or annoying for the

155

victim, the emotions are transient ones and perhaps show as much about the victim's own comfort with genitals as they do about the intent of the flasher. It helps to have a sense of humour.

(If, however, children are the butt of his activities and masturbation is included there is the possibility that this may affect the children's later sexual relationships, although there is no firm evidence to support this at present.) It is really when a flasher is a public nuisance that he needs to be stopped, as much for his own sake as for the people he flashes at.

After-effects of being 'flashed' at appear to be short-lived. No long-term problems have been uncovered as a result of such an experience.

Peeping-toms are another more intrusive type of minor sexual offender in that they are a public nuisance *and* they intrude on people's private activities. If they combine their peeping activities with masturbation, as is common, this in itself is annoying and insulting to victims. They are also usually harmless if unpleasant. Self-help and hospital referral are along the same lines as that suggested for exhibitionists.

TWELVE

Grief and Ageing

The death of a loved relation is a sad and shocking event and most people grieve when a partner, parent or child dies. Grief itself has many forms and how people grieve affects, among many other things, their sex-lives. For example, if the griever is depressed, feelings of sexual desire may disappear. Extreme anger can sometimes slightly unbalance otherwise reasonable people—sexual intercourse being extremely difficult for such angry and obsessed beings.

Grief at the loss of a baby, either 'in utero' or after its birth can alter sexual relations so that they lose their meaning. Grief at the realization that a woman may *never* give birth can have the same effect. Sometimes these sorrows can be selective. After having three sons when she desperately wanted a daughter, one woman passed into a state of grief where she couldn't bear to make love with her husband any more.

Losing a parent can strike at the very foundations of personal security so that even the most seemingly mature 'children' react by withdrawing, avoiding their partner and excusing themselves from making love.

Some women become fixated on a special partner and if he should die or seek divorce, find they are incapable of responding to another, even if they want to. Older women, in particular, may see the death of a partner, as the passing, too, of sexual opportunity and may grieve for their *own sex lives* as well as for their lover. Feeling frozen and set apart are common experiences. So too are interruptions to the menstrual cycle. Some women don't menstruate for months afterward; others experience a painful flooding on the first period after the death.

Getting over grief is a highly individual process. One woman went out as soon as her 32-year-old husband died and sought lovers in case she should lose her nerve altogether. She led a promiscuous lifestyle for about a year before eventually settling down with a second partner. Another, aged forty-nine, went into a depression lasting five years and when she

157

emerged, plunged all her energies into work. She never took up another sexual relationship even though she was able to maintain a sense of humour about this.

Another spent the period immediately after the end of a love affair totally alone. She worked normally during the day but spent most of her evenings locked in the bathroom, crying into the bath. Even though six months later she made a good new relationship, and showed no further outward signs of grief, any difficult emotional situation occurring thereafter threw her back into the grief. It wasn't till she felt she had resolved her sadness ten years later that she firmly committed herself to a permanent sexual relationship once again.

A sixty-year-old grandmother diverted her energies into actively caring for her young grandchildren and made the most of the cuddles and hugs that grandchildren offer. Loving touch, at tragic times, can be a healing factor and just holding someone while they cry, can be a way of allowing them to express their sorrow while feeling supported.

Where the person grieving is an older widow, the realization that loving touch may become a rarity is tragic in itself. Acquiring a furry pet such as a cat, at this stage, may sound simplistic but it is a self-nurturing process. Cuddling and stroking such a pet also gives the stroker good sensations, and these sensual feelings feed into the ego and promote self-confidence.

Recent work by social workers among older people has shown how appreciated massage is when widows (and widowers) have been starved of touch.

The British take a dismissive attitude to old age and sexuality. We could learn a lot from older Americans who have organized networks of friendship, co-operative housing and leisure activities for widows and widowers. It is not unusual there to meet a new partner and remarry in the older age groups and this may reflect something about a particularly American attitude towards enjoying life.

Sex Problems of Grief, and Resolutions

Inability to respond to a new partner

The feeling of being frozen may simply need time in which the

158

psyche can defrost. As a woman gets used to the loss of her former partner she may relax and thaw. However, the ability to express fear and anger can usefully facilitate a 'speeding up' of the grief process. Finding a friend or counsellor with whom to talk on a regular basis is a practical method of working through feelings of sorrow. A caring new partner may help the mourner rebuild an 'inner' platform of trust so that she can relax and experience sexual feeling again.

Inability to feel sexual desire again

Most of the previous paragraph is also true of women who lack sexual desire. If, however, with either problem there seems to be little spontaneous progress towards recovery, this is a signal to seek more specific help either from caring friends or from professional counsellors. It is important to add that even when someone emerges from grief, their life is never going to be quite the same again. One woman, aged forty-nine, recovered quite quickly from intense grief after her husband left her for another woman. She found herself a new and handsome lover with whom she responded easily. But she never felt entirely comfortable with him. This may have been because it can take a very long time to feel mentally separated from a former, deep relationship and therefore at ease with someone new.

Guilt when responding to a new partner

The question of mental separation can do more than make some women feel uncomfortable in new relationships—it can also make them feel guilty. A common experience after widowhood is to feel you are being unfaithful when you are intimate with another partner. The male equivalent of this sensation often results in impotence, and it may be an indication that the individual has not coped adequately with the process of grieving. Perhaps much of the reality of suddenly being alone has been suppressed and, as a result, the quality of ordinary life becomes unreal.

One very good way of working through these feelings is to tackle them as they arise. However hard it may be to do so, opening up about the feelings of guilt to the new partner, seeking their help and understanding, learning to talk and trust, even going through a

type of courtship (which involves taking time over getting to
know each other) assists the new partner to become important
in their own right. This, in turn, helps overcome sadness about
the old one. The use of massage and self-pleasuring exercises
may assist the process (see Appendix 1).

It may help also, to realize that the deceased would not wish a
loved partner to endure unnecessary loneliness—perhaps for
many years. In fact, it is a tribute to that former partnership if
the survivor wishes to recapture the feelings of loving and
sharing a second, or even third time around.

Loneliness leading to unsuitable, incompatible relationships

Establishing networks of friends, acquiring a pet to cuddle and
stroke, going back to work if you are not already there, all
provide forms of companionship. If, in this way, it is possible to
establish an inner security, the widowed or divorced woman is
in a stronger position to choose a new partner rather than opt
for the first available one.

There is no cure for incompatibility and learning to look after
yourself, rather than cling on to the first man who is supposed
to take care of you but doesn't, is a healthy method of
combating loneliness.

Anger or feeling of 'rejection'

If after death or divorce a woman becomes and remains
permanently angry with men it indicates she has got stuck
halfway through the grieving process. Before she can relax and
see men as vulnerable human beings like herself, she needs to
become 'unstuck'. Although it is possible to manage this with
the passing of time and caring friends, it's hard to do so without
some structured help. A therapist for example, enables such a
'stuck' mourner to *experience her anger more fully*, and thus *facilitate
her further through the stages of grief*.

Sex problems of age

Dyspareunia

As fully discussed in the section on the menopause (Chapter 6)
the withdrawal of the hormone oestrogen from the body, after

the menopause, can cause a gradual drying of vaginal tissue, with the result that intercourse may become painful. Hormone therapy will overcome this problem where it is severe. Oestrogen cream, applied locally, will also be helpful. (See Chapters 4 and 6 for details.)

Diminished sexual desire

Some women experience a general lessening of interest in sex as they grow older. Surveys of the sexuality of older women find that although sexual interest persists after the menopause, it diminishes in many women after the age of sixty. Yet there is such emphasis laid on sex in our culture that we are brainwashed into thinking there is something wrong with older women who are no longer strongly motivated sexually. It is important to get it clear that there are real reasons why this is *not* the case.

As individuals we vary. Just as some little girls are sexy, so too are some older women. The majority of us fit into the 'average' state where, in general, sex is very pleasant providing it works well. This applies to sex after sixty too. If you are lucky enough to remain in a caring and sexually successful relationship the odds are that sex will remain a caring experience despite increasing age. There just may not be so much of it. If, however, sex has been unsatisfactory for years or if it has never been interesting for you—or if you have learned to live without sex because you have lived without a partner—the odds are sex will take a very low key role in your old age. But this in no way diminishes the personality. We are still full of enjoyment and purpose. We do not diminish as people because our sexual desire changes. Do not let anyone convince you otherwise.

To get present-day expectations of sex and age completely in proportion it is useful to compare youth and old age. Just as it is a myth to think we must all be sexy until we're 100, it is also a myth to think that all small children are devoid of sexuality. It may suit us to think so but it isn't actually the case. However, we don't expect young children to have active sex lives because there are good physiological reasons why this is undesirable. Why, therefore, do we expect all older women to remain sexual when there are physiological reasons why this is no longer sensible? Sex for older women is highly variable and reflects circumstances rather than inadequate personality.

The real sex problems of age arise if and when we meet a new partner after having adapted to the more celibate situation of widowhood. Should it prove impossible to muster sexual interest, one option is to agree that the emphasis in the relationship will be on companionship rather than on sex. Another is to agree to be a willing if passive partner. A third is to seek hormonal help to facilitate a return of sexual interest and response.

The most unexpected candidates are capable of discovering a full sex life. One of my oldest clients was an 85-year-old who had married for the first time three years previously to a man who was extremely interested in sex. When she explained that she had a few problems with discomfort it became quickly apparent that there wasn't much wrong with her sexual response—it was just that her husband wanted sex every night!

It may seem crude to some, when discussing grief and old age, to write about masturbation and sex aids such as KY jelly. But the need to relieve sexual frustration, the need to seek personal sexual comfort and the need to facilitate intercourse are all true of older grieving people just as they are of anyone else.

Masturbation may be instrumental in keeping alive a woman's sense of her own sexuality and therefore of her sexual identity during widowhood and old age. It may also be responsible for keeping her physiological sexual responses in 'good working order'. The ability to use this relief and comfort may prevent a lonely woman from making an unsuitable new alliance and allow her to re-arrange her social life from a position of choice rather than need.

In a new relationship where response may be hampered by the ageing process, using a little KY jelly or even Orthogynal jelly, could make all the difference.

Life expectation being what it is, it is a fair guess that most of the women reading this book will end up being widows. While, of course, the period of transition between our former married lives and our newer single lives is painful, it is worth keeping a firm eye on the fact that many of us go on to lead rich, full lives afterwards—even if they are altered ones.

Conclusion

The emphasis throughout the book has been on self-help and the appendices include methods and programmes of sexual self-help exercises. But the body isn't a machine and sexual response is as much an element of thought as it is of physiological reflex.

In plain terms this means that the mind can get in the way of the most well meaning exercises and sabotage them. No therapy, be it self-help or professional, can have a successful outcome until the reasons for the sabotage have been sorted out and dealt with, thus enabling the saboteur to get past a mental block.

Some people are born with an instinctive skill in working out their own problems and helping others to do likewise. They will probably find sex therapy exercises easy and the marital discussion stimulating. Others are not so fortunate, they need to acquire the skills and self-help may not be enough.

Hopefully, it will have become clear by now that sex therapy is not the simplistic technical science it once purported to be. Most so-called sex problems are not just sex problems, they are social and psychological ones. If someone is wounded deep in the subconscious as a child, it shows in their ability (or lack of it) to make a satisfactory relationship. Perhaps the sexual side of the relationship throws up shadows of the wound or perhaps the rest of the sufferer's psyche is so darkened that their feeling of worthlessness spreads to and includes their sex life.

Outside pressures cannot be discounted. We are all moulded to fit the society we are born in to. Yet some of us don't want to get married, have children, be fat, thin, have big breasts or small. How we balance our gut feelings versus the wishes of our parents are only two of the complicating factors that influence our happiness.

For those who have gained insight into their problems by reading this book but seem to be unable to get very far in solving them on their own the next step is to seek outside help. It needs to be the right outside help. Sometimes one counsellor may be inadequate—this is not, however, an indication that all counsellors are. Like any other profession, counsellors specialize in certain problems and certain methods of therapy. A good counsellor will be able to acknowledge his or her limitations and will recommend someone who can take the client further.

Part of the counselling process is also to distinguish those clients who will benefit from simple counselling and/or simple sex therapy from those who need the 'in-depth' help of psychotherapy. Medical screening for any entrenched sex problem is a must, too, and if there is any hint that the problem may be caused for organic reasons, specific medical referral ought to be made, if only to eliminate medical causes. It stands to reason that years of counselling will get nowhere if someone's hormone balance is so askew it has deprived them of physical sensation. All these investigations take time and require patience.

Starting points for sex therapy may be the doctor, or the marriage guidance counsellor, or a local counselling advisory service. Specific help can be sought from:
- Sex therapy clinics.
- The Association of Marital and Sexual Therapists and psychosexual units in the main teaching hospitals. Not all psychosexual units need doctors' referral—it is sometimes possible to refer yourself.
- Many excellent private therapists operate as marriage counsellors and sex therapists; some work within a clinic, others in a private practice. Appendix 2 gives a list of sources of free psycho-sexual counselling.
- There are also many self-help groups for special problems that do invaluable work in support work, counselling, information gathering and dissemination. A good and reliable referral source for these is *The Sunday Times Self-Help Directory* which lists hundreds of names, addresses and details of services.

Anyone who fears a professional helper will 'tell' you what to do can relax. A counsellor helps *you* to make decisions and is not in the position of taking them for you. The best kind of counsellor will assist you to marry up that 'inner' woman with the outer one. It can be a fascinating process.

Appendices

APPENDIX ONE

Sex Therapy Self-Help Programmes

Self-pleasuring routine for women only

Based on methods used by the Women's Sexuality Workshop in pre-orgasmic groups, this is a special programme of 'erotic homework' to be carried out in the privacy of your own room. You may take six days over it or six weeks; it is important to feel comfortable and unhurried. If you find yourself 'sabotaging' the sessions, it means you have gone too far too fast. You need to return to a previous step.

Preparations

Ensure there is privacy. If necessary fit a bolt to the door of your room. All self-massage should be carried out in a warm atmosphere and it is sensible to heat the room in advance. When applying massage oil to yourself, never drop the oil directly on to your skin from the bottle. Always smooth it on lightly with your hands. Try to ensure the oil and your hands are warm.

1   After relaxing in a hot bath, apply the warmed oil (you can float the bottle in the bath to warm it up) all over your body. The oil should be sweet smelling and preferably appeal to your sensuality. Massage yourself sensitively, oiling the skin everywhere except the genitals. The aim is to discover which parts of your body feel sensual and which do not.

2   Repeat this routine, only including the genitals. Each stage should be confined to one session only.

3   Repeat again, concentrating more on the genitals and less on the body.

4   Explore the genitals more fully, not with orgasm as an aim, but simply in order to re-awaken good feelings.

5   Repeat no 4 taking it further. Build on the good sensations you get from stroking your breasts, your stomach, thighs, genitals, anywhere which gives good feeling. Build on the feelings of excitement generated from this. If you feel yourself

approaching orgasm, continue the stimulation and see what happens. (It doesn't matter if you don't climax, the object of this exercise is to explore all erotic sensation.)

Every woman stimulates herself in a way that is uniquely her own. Some women stimulate the whole of their genitals and not the clitoris alone. This takes longer to lead to excitement but turns arousal into a powerfully exciting experience. Others prefer concentrating a very light touch on the clitoris alone, such as fingertip twirling. Some people prefer stimulating only one side of the clitoral shaft, and if orgasm does happen, stimulation needs to continue until the climax is completed. It doesn't carry on, on its own, without continued stimulation.

If, at any time, such stimulation becomes dry and painful, this may mean more massage oil is needed. If lubrication is not the problem, but the stimulation grows uncomfortable, try focusing on erotic fantasy or sexy thoughts to lift your body above the anxiety you are feeling which is responsible for the discomfort.
6   (Optional) Don't persevere too long on no 5 if this proves frustrating. No 6 is much the same as no 5 only instead of fingers, use a vibrator. Vibrators sometimes provide more stimulation than fingers can, either because their movement is more rapid or because they are *not* actually part of your body.

This brief version of the Women's Sexuality Workshop self-pleasuring programme aims to re-awaken sensation or to build up for the first time sensation which will provide sensual feeling and eventually orgasm. For fuller details of the programme, please see *The Body Electric* by Anne Hooper (Unwin Paperbacks).

Self-pleasuring routine for couples when the woman has not yet experienced orgasm

This routine is based on methods used by Masters and Johnson. The pre-requisites of warm room, massage oil and agreement to work over a number of weeks are the same as in the previous pre-orgasmic routine. You may take as many weeks as you feel necessary for these exercises and any time you feel uncomfortable with what you are doing, go back a step. Intercourse is forbidden until specified.

The aim here is not only to re-awaken your sexual feeling,

but also to encourage the growth of trust and communication between you and your partner. In order to facilitate this it is necessary that you both learn to exchange information about giving and receiving sensual touch. Your partner should ask for feedback about the effectiveness of his touch, you should contribute this voluntarily. Feedback doesn't have to mean a solemn rating; it can consist of groans, grunts and cries of ecstasy! When something feels specially good, tell your partner so that he can learn to build on that. When a touch needs to be altered slightly, ask for the alteration. In this way you will both learn to communicate about intimate touch.

1 Share a warm bath together, slowly and sensuously soaping each other all over, excluding the genitals. Then transfer from the bathroom to a heated room where you can carry out a mutual massage. You should massage him first, then he massages you. The object of this exercise is to discover each other's erogenous zones and to build up a picture of each other's 'body map'. The genitals are not massaged on this first occasion. Each of you should let the other know when their touch is effective and when it is not. The whole of the body area can be massaged. Each massage should take at least twenty minutes, or more. At this stage, the massage is carried out with each partner lying down.
2 The warm bath and massage are repeated as in step 1 only this time the genitals are included in the massage. They should be treated in the same way as the rest of the body. They are being explored to obtain information about their sensitivity and the exchange of information concerning the effectiveness of the massage should continue just as it has for the rest of the massage. The genitals are *not* being massaged in order to obtain orgasm.
3 This time, after the warm bath, the routine alters. When it is your turn, to be massaged, after your body has been massaged you should both alter your position. He leans back against some pillows in a sitting position while you seat yourself between his legs, leaning against him. Your back is resting against his chest. He can hold you with tenderness while positioning his other hand between your legs. In this way you will be able to place one hand over his so that you can influence the way in which he touches you. Now he explores your genitals in much the same

manner as in the previous phase, starting with the insides of the thighs, going on to the external genitalia and progressing to the inner labia and the clitoris. The exploration is done as a sensitive massage and you give him feedback on the quality of his touch just as you did previously. This is the time to explore different areas of sensitivity, different types of touch, pressure and movement.

4   Repeat no 4, spending more time and discussion on the genitals and building on what have been reported as the more sensual sensations. If necessary you may show your man which types of touch feel good, or may take control of his caressing hand. If the progress of these strokes is impeded by lack of lubrication your partner may either gently insert his finger into your vagina and spread some of your natural lubrication on to your genitals, or he may use the massage oil as a logical extension of the massage. The purpose of this exercise is to give you the chance of concentrating on your own sexual feelings.

5   When you report pleasurable and intense sexual sensation (this might have included orgasm but it doesn't matter if it didn't) the exercise shifts to intercourse with your man lying on his back and you kneeling over him in order to insert his penis. (This of course only takes place after the massage exercise of the previous stage and not 'cold'.) To begin with you must hold still on your partner's penis and just appreciate containing him. You may practise tightening and relaxing your vaginal muscles and both of you can focus on the sensations in your genitals.

6   At the next session the same procedure is fulfilled, only this time you may carry out some brief thrusting.

7   At each subsequent session the thrusting may become longer. The intercourse is still practised without a climax as an aim. Once you feel open to the sensation provided by thrusting you may discover you can climax anyhow. The process is a gradual one and takes time.

8   (Optional) Some couples reach an extremely sensual stage of intercourse but do not, nevertheless, receive quite enough sensation via intercourse only to encourage orgasm. In this case, experimentation with fingers, or different positions or the addition of a vibrator often help you both to enjoy climax.

Because these exercises are carried out in the context of a relationship there may be hidden fears and resentments which get in the way of actually carrying out the routine. Please see Chapters 1 and 2 for further details. As a matter of principle, talking about and attempting to resolve the difficult emotions therapy can throw up, go a long way to contributing towards the trust and appreciation needed for the success of these exercises.

More details of couples' sexual exercises to improve both intercourse and verbal communication may be found in *Treat Yourself to Sex* by Paul Brown and Carolyn Faulder (Penguin).

How to use a speculum

Assemble together a large mirror, tissues, KY jelly, a bright light and disposable speculum. Lubricate the speculum with the KY jelly.

The best position in which to insert the speculum is while half-sitting, half lying, propped against cushions. The speculum blades are held together to avoid pinching the wall of the vagina during entry and insertion takes place with the handle held upwards. Take your time over the insertion, there is no hurry and if any panic is experienced just pause and breathe deeply till you get used to the sensation and can continue. After insertion has gone as far as you feel comfortable with, the handle can be squeezed gently so that the ratchet opens the blades.

While you are doing this, watch your progress in the mirror which has been propped in front of you and by courtesy of the bright light which you should angle to give the maximum view to your vagina.

The speculum can be opened one notch at a time until your cervix is visible. According to the textbooks, the cervix lies directly at the back of the vaginal opening. In fact, it can be located at a variety of angles, and you may have to move the speculum around cautiously until the cervix and the os (the tiny opening in the cervix) comes into sight. When you have finished viewing, the speculum can be removed by pulling it slowly but firmly from the vagina. It is not necessary to close it first.

Since it is complicated to juggle with speculum, light and mirror simultaneously, it is helpful if the first couple of times you practise this, you do so with the aid of a supportive friend.

Speculae may be obtained from surgical suppliers, whose

names are usually listed in the yellow pages telephone directory.

Further information on the use of a speculum and how to understand what you see may be found in *The Body Electric* by Anne Hooper (Unwin Paperbacks).

APPENDIX TWO

Recommended Reading and Helping Agencies

PART 1: PROBLEMS OF SEXUAL RESPONSE

Sex Education: Recommended reading
Make It Happy by Jane Cousins (Penguin)
  A sex education book for teenagers.
How a Baby is Made by Per-Holm Knudsen (Piccolo)
  A picture story with simple text of the facts of life.

Educational counselling
Brook Advisory Centres (all over the country)
Head Office
153a East Street,
London SE17
(01 708 1234)

Family Planning Association (provides counselling in some areas)
Head Office
27–35 Mortimer Street,
London W1N 7RJ
(01 636 7866)

Women's Sex Problems: Recommended reading

The Body Electric by Anne Hooper (Unwin Paperbacks)
  Fictional account of a sexuality group for women with details
  of the pre-orgasmic programme used for self-help.
Total Orgasm by Jack Lee Rosenberg, (Wildwood House, 1974)
  Bioenergetic exercise and philosophy.

Pre-orgasmic groups
Some hospitals run women's sexuality groups within their
psychosexual unit (usually attached to a medical school). A
telephone call to the hospital should let you know if a group
exists and whether or not you need GP referral. See list of
general addresses for psycho-sexual counselling. One-to-one

counselling may be available for individual women with sex problems.

Spare Rib magazine
Lists women's self-help groups and may include sexuality groups.

Women's Sexuality Workshop
58 The Pryors,
East Heath Road,
London NW3
Runs pre-orgasmic groups three times a year.

Redwood
83 Fordych Road,
London NW2
Runs a variety of programmes concerning sex problems and assertion training.

London Institute for the Study of Human Sexuality
10 Warwick Road,
London SW5
Provides counselling for most aspects of sexual health.

Women's Therapy Centre
6 Manor Gardens,
London N7
Provides psycho-therapy and specialist workshops on aspects of sexuality, body image, assertion, etc.

Self-help
For details of how to start your own pre-orgasmic self-help group see *The Body Electric* by Anne Hooper (Unwin)

Body Image: Recommended reading
Fat is a Feminist Issue by Susie Orbach (Hamlyn Paperbacks)
The Art of Starvation by Sheila Macleod (Virago)

Body image groups
Women's Therapy Centre
6 Manor Gardens,
London N7
Runs groups for women with eating problems. Compulsive eating groups are set up on a self-help basis around the country. To get in touch with these, contact your local women's organiz-

ations for names and addresses. Citizens Advice Bureaux should be able to put you in touch with the women's organizations. CAB is in the telephone directory.

Assertion training
Redwood,
83 Fordwych Road,
London NW2
Offers assertion training.

LifeSkills,
3 Brighton Road,
London N2
Offers assertion training.
Some local authorities now run assertion training groups for women and local authority information centres would advise. Local women's centres would also have details of local assertion training.

Recommended reading
A Woman in Her Own Right by Anne Dickson (Quartet)
LifeSkills 1: Assertiveness by Robert Sharpe (Behavioural Press)

Career counselling
Frederick Chusid,
35 Fitzroy Street,
London W1
Has other regional branches.

Contraceptive advice
Family Planning Association
Head Office,
27–35 Mortimer Street,
London W1
Has offices all over the country. Details in the local telephone directory.

Brook Advisory Centres
Head Office,
153a East Street,
London SE 17
Have offices all over the country. Details in local telephone directory.

Recommended reading
A variety of texts is available from both the above organizations
and the Family Planning Association has a Book Sales department from which a catalogue is obtainable.

Marital problems: Recommended reading
Treat Yourself to Sex by Paul Brown and Carolyn Faulder (Penguin)
  Discusses common marital sex problems and provides sex
  therapy methods for self-help.
Marriage and How To Survive It by Dougal Mackay and Jill Frankham
(Piatkus Books)
  Advice on how to work on marriage problems.
Women and Depression by Deidre Sanders (Sheldon Press)
  A practical self-help guide.

Marriage counselling
Marriage Guidance Council have offices all over the country.
Addresses in local telephone directory.

CHAPTER TWO: LACK OF DESIRE

Lack of Desire: Recommended reading
Disorders of Sexual Desire by Helen Singer Kaplan (Balliere Tindall)
  Text for sex therapy students and practitioners.
  See list of addresses for sex therapy counselling.

Surrogate therapy
The Institute of Sex Education and Research
38 School Road,
Moseley,
Birmingham 13
(021 449 0892)

Vibrators
On sale at most large chemists or by mail order from certain
suppliers. See *She* or *Forum* magazines for up-to-date details of
suppliers.

CHAPTER THREE: DIFFICULTIES WITH MASTURBATION

Masturbation: Recommended reading

Orgasm and Self-Love by Betty Dodson (formerly titled *Liberating Masturbation* (Bodysex Designs) available mail order only from Marriage Guidance Mail Order Book Sales, Herbert Gray College, Little Church Street, Rugby, Warks for £3.75 plus 30 pence p&p.

The Body Electric by Anne Hooper (Unwin Paperbacks) See page 173 for details of pre-orgasmic groups and page 191 for lists of counselling addresses.

CHAPTER FOUR: PAINFUL SEX

Advice

Any pain should be presented to the GP for diagnosis. If necessary he or she will refer you on to a specialist department at the nearest large hospital. See next section for VD addresses.

CHAPTER FIVE: SEXUAL DISEASES

VD Clinics

Specialist advice can be obtained at the Special Clinics or VD Clinics which are situated in all the main large hospitals. Doctor's referral is *not* needed. Hospitals' addresses and telephone numbers in telephone directory.

Recommended reading
Cystitis by Angela Kilmartin (Arrow)
Thrush by Caroline Clayton (Sheldon Press)
Herpes By Dr J. K. Oates (Penguin)

Self-help
Simplex
PO Box 59
London WC1X 0LD
(01 833 4467)
Provides information and social contact for herpes sufferers.

The Terence Higgins Trust
(01 833 2971)
  Provides support for people with AIDS and information about the syndrome.

CHAPTER SIX: HORMONES A ND SEX

PMT: Recommended reading
Understanding Premenstrual Tension by Dr Michael Brush (Pan)
  The most up-to-date book presently available.

Clinical advice
Many of the larger teaching hospitals hold clinics for women with PMT problems, often in association with their menopause clinics. Doctor's referral is generally needed.

The Pre-Menstrual Tension Advisory Service
PO Box 268,
Hove
East Sussex BN3 1RW
(0273 771366)
  Provides diagnosis, advice and nutritional supplement

Post-Natal Depression: Recommended reading
Post-Natal Depression by Vivienne Welburn (Fontana)

Counselling and advice
National Childbirth Trust,
9 Queensborough Terrace,
London W2
(01 229 9319)

Association for Postnatal Illness
7 Gowan Avenue,
London SW6

Menopause: Recommended reading
No Change by Wendy Cooper (Arrow)

Counselling and advice
All except one of the hospitals and institutions listed below

offer NHS clinics. Referral should be through your own GP in the first instance; the usual department is 'Gyn and Obst'.

Aberdeen	Gynaecology and Endocrine Clinic, Aberdeen University, Foresthill
Belfast	Samaritan Hospital, Lisburn Road, Belfast
Birmingham	Women's Hospital, Professorial Unit, Queen Elizabeth Medical Centre, Edgbaston, Birmingham B15 2TG
Brighton	Royal Sussex Hospital, Brighton, Sussex
Bristol	Southmead Hospital, Westbury-on-Trym
—	Royal Infirmary, Bristol
Beckenham	Beckenham Hospital, 279 Croydon Road, Beckenham, Kent
Dublin	Coombe Hospital, Dublin 8
Durham	Dryburn Hospital, Durham
Edinburgh	Royal Infirmary, 39 Chalmers Street, Edinburgh EH3 9ER
Glasgow	Glasgow Royal Infirmary, Menopause Clinic, Castle Street, G4 0SF
—	Glasgow Western Infirmary, Dunbarton Road, G11
—	Stobhill Hospital, Balornock Road, G21
Hove	The Lady Chichester Hospital, New Church Street, Hove, Sussex
Leeds	Women's Hospital, Leeds
Liverpool	Women's Hospital, Gynaecological Unit, Catherine Street, Liverpool
London	Chelsea Hospital for Women, Dovehouse Street, SW3
—	Dulwich Hospital, East Dulwich Grove, SE21
—	King's College Hospital, Denmark Hill, SE5
—	St George's Hospital, Blackshaw Road, Tooting, SW17
—	St Thomas's Hospital, SE1
—	Samaritan Hospital for Women, Marylebone Road, NW1
—	Royal Free Hospital, Pond Street, NW3
—	Soho Hospital for Women, Soho Square, W1
Manchester	Wythenshaw Hospital, Southmoor Road, Manchester 22
—	Manchester General Hospital, Crumpsall, Manchester M8 6RB
Newcastle	Newcastle General Hospital, Westgate Road, Newcastle-upon-Tyne, NE4 6BE

Nuneaton	George Elliot Hospital, College Street, Nuneaton, Warwickshire
Oxford	The John Radcliffe Hospital, Oxford
Peterborough	Peterborough and District Hospital, Thorpe Road, Peterborough
Rotherham	Menopause Clinic, Moorgate General Hospital, Rotherham, Yorkshire
Sheffield	Royal Hallamshire Hospital, Glossop Road, Sheffield S10 2JF
Stafford	Stafford General Infirmary, Stafford
Staines	Ashford Hospital, Staines, Middlesex
Stockport	Stepping Hill Hospital, Stockport, Cheshire
Wales	Simbech Research Centre, Merthyr Tydfil (not NHS but a *free* clinic.)

CHAPTER SEVEN: PREGNANCY AND SEXUAL RESPONSE

Pregnancy: Recommended reading
The Experience of Childbirth by Sheila Kitzinger (Penguin)

Infertility: Recommended reading
Why Us? by Dr Andrew Stanway (Granada)
Overcoming Childlessness by Elliot Philipp (Hamlyn)
Coping with Childlessness by Diane and Peter Houghton (George Allen and Unwin)

Self-help
The National Association for the Childless,
Birmingham Settlement,
318 Summer Lane,
Birmingham, B19 3RL

CHAPTER NINE: ILLNESS AND SEXUALITY

Self-help
HEART ATTACK
Chest, Heart and Stroke Association,
Tavistock House North,
Tavistock Square,
London WC1H 9JE
(01 387 3012)
   Registered charity working to help people affected by chest, heart and stroke illnesses.

Scotland
65 North Castle Street,
Edinburgh, EH2 3LT
(031 225 6527)

N. Ireland
28 Bedford Street,
Belfast BT2 7FJ
Belfast 20184

Cardiac Spare Parts,
10 Duke Street,
Little Common,
Bexhill-on-Sea,
East Sussex
  A mutual aid society for people who have undergone or
  require major heart surgery.

HYPERTENSION
Hypertensives Register,
Ms Cass McCallum,
Errol,
Perth,
Scotland.
  Personal counselling on hypertension and drug treatment.
  Send sae when writing for information.

DIABETES
British Diabetic Association,
10 Queen Anne Street,
London W1M 0BD
(01 323 1531)

RENAL FAILURE
British Kidney Patient Association,
Bordon, Hants
Bordon 2021/2

ARTHRITIS
Arthritis Care,
6 Grosvenor Crescent,
London SE1
(01 235 0902)
  Offers information, advice and practical aid.

MULTIPLE SCLEROSIS
Multiple Sclerosis Society of Great Britain and Northern Ireland,
286 Munster Road,
London SW6
(01 381 4022/5)

STROKE
See heart section

EPILEPSY
British Epilepsy Association,
Crowthorne House,
Bigshotte,
New Wokingham Road,
Wokingham, Berks RG11 3AY
Crowthorne 3122

SPINAL INJURIES
Spinal Injuries Association,
5 Crowndale Road,
London NW1 1TU
(01 388 6840)

ILEOSTOMY
Ileostomy Association of Great Britain and Ireland,
Amblehurst House,
Chobham,
Woking,
Surrey GU24 8PZ
Chobham 8277

MASTECTOMY
Mastectomy Association,
1 Colworth Road,
Croydon,
Surrey
(01 654 8643)

Mastectomy Centre,
12 Henrietta Place,
London W1
(01 580 1602)

RADIOTHERAPY
Marie Curie Memorial Foundation,
124 Sloane Street,
London SW1X 9BP
(01 730 9157)

PSYCHOLOGICAL ILLNESS: *Recommended reading*
  The Family Doctor Publications group publish a variety of
  inexpensive and informative booklets on aspects of illness
  and surgery. A list of these is available on receipt of an sae.
  Family Doctor Publications,
  British Medical Association,
  Tavistock Square,
  London WC1H 9JP

EATING DISORDERS: *Recommended reading*
Anorexia: *The Art of Starvation* by Sheila Macleod (Virago)
Bulimia: *A Glutton for Punishment* by Louise Roche (Pan)

DEPRESSION: *Recommended reading*
Women and Depression by Deidre Sanders (Sheldon Press)
Depression—A Way Out of the Prison by Dorothy Rowe (RKP)
Depression: Why It Happens and How to Overcome It by Dr Paul Hauck
  (Sheldon Press)

Addresses
MIND (National Association for Mental Health)
22 Harley Street,
London W1N 2ED
  The leading mental health association in England and Wales.
  It supplies information and expertise to people with mental
  problems.

CHAPTER TEN: LESBIANISM

LESBIANISM: *Recommended reading*
Our Right to Love: a lesbian resource book edited by Ginny Vida (New
  Jersey: Prentice-Hall Inc)
Sappho was a Right-on Woman by Sidney Abbott and Barbara Love
  (Stein and Day)
  There are many other texts available on lesbianism. Com-

pendium Bookshop, 240 Camden High Street, London NW1
supplies a list on receipt of an sae.

Self-help
Gemma
BM 5700,
London WC1N 3XX
For lesbians with and without disabilities, to lessen social
isolation.

Kenric
BM Kenric,
London WC1N 3XX
International, non-political organization for gay women,
social activities in London area.

For lesbian social groups in areas other than London the
following telephone numbers of women-only switchboards
will provide up-to-date details.

England
Birmingham *lesbian line* Mon., Weds. 7–10pm (021) 622 6580
Bradford *lesbian line* Thurs. 7–9pm (0274) 305525
Cambridge *lesbian line switchboard* Fri. 6–10pm (0223) 346113
Colchester *lesbian line* Weds. 8–10pm (0206) 870051
Coventry *lesbian line* Weds. 7–10pm (0203) 77105
Lancaster *women's line* Wed. 2–9pm (0524) 63021
Leeds *lesbian nightline* Tues. 7.30–9.30pm (0532) 453588
Liverpool *women's line* Tues. and Thurs. 7.30–10.00pm (051) 708
234
London *lesbian line* Mon. and Fri. 2–10pm (01) 251 6911
London *Friend women's line* Thurs. 7.30–10pm (01) 354 6305
Manchester *lesbian line* Mon. to Fri. 7–10pm (061) 2366305
Newcastle *lesbian line* Thurs., Fri. 7–10pm (0632) 612277
North Staffs *lesbian support group* Fri. 7–10pm (0782) 266998
Norwich *lesbian line* Weds. 8–10pm (0603) 628055
Nottingham *lesbian line* Mon., Weds. 7–9.30pm (0602) 410652
Oxford *lesbian line* Weds. 7–10pm (0865) 242333
Preston *lesbian line* Mon. and Wed. 8–9.30pm (0772) 51122
Reading *lesbian helpline* Tues., Friday 8–10pm (0734) 597269
Sheffield *lesbian line* Thurs. 7–10pm (0742) 581238
Ireland
Belfast *Carafriend* Thurs. 8–10pm (0232) 22023

Dublin NFG *Switchboard* Thurs. 8–10pm (01) 71 06 08
IRGM Munster Cork Thurs. 8–10pm (021) 505 394
Scotland
Aberdeen *lesbian line* Wed. 7–10pm (0224) 572726
Dundee *lesbian line* Tues. 7–10pm (0382) 21843
Edinburgh *(Scottish young lesbian line)* Mon. and Wed. 8–10pm (031) 557 3620
Glasgow *lesbian line* Mon. 7–10pm (041) 248 4596
Wales
Cardiff *lesbian line* Thurs. 8–10pm (0222) 374051
Swansea *lesbian line* Fri. 7–10pm (0792) 467 365

Parents Enquiry,
Rose Robertson,
16 Honley Road,
London SE6 2HZ
(01 698 1815)
Counselling organization for homosexual teenagers and their families.

Redwood,
83 Fordwych Road,
London NW2
Assertion training for women with local branches all over the country. Send sae for national details.

National Association for the Childless,
Birmingham Settlement,
318 Summer Lane,
Birmingham B19 3RL
(021-359-4887/2113/3563)
Self-help group to provide support and counselling for people undergoing fertility treatment and for the childless.

Lesbian Mothers Group,
c/o The Gay Centre,
61a Bloom Street,
Manchester.

Sexual information
The G-Spot, by Ladas, Whipple and Perry (Corgi)

CHAPTER ELEVEN: RAPE, INCEST AND EXHIBITIONISM

Rape

Rape crisis centres

Aberdeen	P.O. Box 123, Aberdeen. *Tel.* 0224 575560 Mon. 6–8pm; Thurs. 7–9pm
Belfast	P.O. Box 46, Belfast BT2 7AR. *Tel.* 0232 249696 Tues. and Fri. 7–10pm
Birmingham	P.O. Box 558, Birmingham B3 2HL. *Tel.* 021 233 2122. Office 021 233 2655 24hrs, 7 days a week
Bradford	c/o 31 Manor Row, Bradford, West Yorks. *Tel.* 0274 308270. Mon. 1–5pm; Thurs. 6–10pm
Brighton	P.O. Box 232, Hove, E. Sussex BN3 3XB. *Tel.* 0273 699756 Tues. 6–9pm; Fri. 3–9pm; Sat. 10am–1pm
Bristol	(Incest Survivors project as well) 39 Jamaica Street, Bristol 2. *Tel.* 0272 428331. Mon.–Fri. 10.30am–2.30pm
Cambridge	Box R.12, Mill Road, Cambridge. *Tel.* 0223 358314 Wed. 6–12pm; Sat. 11am–5pm
Central Scotland	P.O. Box 4, Falkirk. *Tel.* 0324 38433 Mon. and Thurs. 7–9pm
Chelmsford	c/o 42 Darnay Rise, Melbourne, Chelmsford, Essex
Cleveland	P.O. Box 31, Middlesbrough, Cleveland, TS4 2JJ. *Tel.* 0642 225787. Mon.–Wed. 10am–3pm; Thurs. 10am–3pm and 7–10pm
Cork	P.O. Box 42, Brian Boru Street, Cork, Eire. *Tel.* 021 0002 968086 Mon. 7.30–10pm; Wed. 2–5pm; Fri. 10am–1pm; Sat. 1–4pm
Coventry	P.O. Box 176, Coventry CV1 2OS. *Tel.* 0203 77229 Mon. 11–3pm; 7–10pm; Tues.–Fri. 11am–3pm
Cumbria	P.O. Box 21, Kendal, Cumbria LA9 4BU. *Tel.* 0539 25255. Mon. 7–10pm; Wed. 12am–3pm
Canterbury	*Tel.* 0227 450400. Every evening 6pm–9pm
Derby	c/o Women's centre, the Guildhall, Derby. *Tel.* 0332 372545. Thurs. 7.30–9.30pm
Dublin	P.O. Box 1027, Dublin 6, Eire. *Tel.* 01-0001 601470 Mon.–Fri. 8am–8pm; Sat.–Sun. 24hr
Edinburgh	P.O. Box 120, Edinburgh, E11 3ND. *Tel.* 031 556 9437 Mon. and Wed. 1–2pm, 6–8pm; Thurs. 7–10pm; Fri. 6–8pm
Exeter	c/o Pennsylvania Road, Exeter. *Tel.* 0392 30871 24hr, 7 days a week
Galway, Eire	*Tel.* 091 66747

Gloucester	Russet House, Russet Close, Tuffley, Gloucester-shire. *Tel.* 0452 26770 Mon. 7.30–9.30pm; Thurs. 11.30–2pm
Highlands	c/o 38 Ardonnell Street, Inverness. *Tel.* 0463 220719 Mon., Thurs., Sat., Sun. 7–10pm
Hull	P.O. Box 40, Hull, Humberside. *Tel.* 0482 29990 Thurs. 4–12pm
Leamington	Box 22, 12 Gloucester Street, Leamington Spa. *Tel.* 0926 832529 Tues. 7.30–10pm
Grays Thurrock (Essex)	Bridge House, Bridge Road, Grays Thurrock. *Tel.* 0375 38609 Mon. 6–9pm; Wed. 1–5pm; Tues. 7pm–10pm; Thurs. 12 noon–4pm
Leeds	P.O. Box 27, Leeds LS2 7EG. *Tel.* 0532 440058 10am–Midnight every day
Leicester	70 High Street, Leicester. *Tel.* 0533 666666 Tues. 7–10pm; Sat. 2–5pm
Limerick	P.O. Box 128, Limerick, Eire. *Tel.* 061 41211
Liverpool	P.O. Box 64, Liverpool L69 8AT Mon. 7–9pm; Thurs. and Sat. 2–5pm
London	RCRP, P.O. Box 69, London WC1X 9NJ 24hr, 7 days a week. *Tel.* 01 837 1600
Luton	12 Oxford Road, Luton. *Tel.* (office) 0582 33426 (helpline) 0582 33592 Mon.–Fri. 9am–5pm; Mon. 7–10pm; Wed. 7–10pm
Manchester	P.O. Box 336, Manchester M60 2BS. *Tel.* 061 228 3602 Tues. and Fri. 2–5pm; Wed., Thurs., Sun. 6–9pm
Milton Keynes	The Bakehouse, and Church Street, Wolverton, Milton Keynes, Bucks
Nottingham	37a Mansfield Road, Nottingham. *Tel.* 0602 410440 Tues.–Fri. 10am–4pm; Sat. 10am–1pm
Norwich	P.O. Box 47, Norwich, NR1 2BU. *Tel.* 0603 667687 Mon. 6–8pm; Fri. 11am–2pm; Thurs. 8–10pm; Sat. 4–6pm
Oxford (Women's Line)	P.O. Box 73, Oxford OX3 6ET. *Tel.* 0865 726295 Wed. 2–10pm
Plymouth	c/o Box A, Virginia House, Palace Street, Plymouth, PL4 0EQ *Tel.* 0752 23584. Thurs. 7.30–10pm
Portsmouth	P.O. Box 3, Southsea, Portsmouth PO4 9FC. *Tel.* 0705 669511 Wed. and Sat. 7–10pm; Fri. 7pm–7am; Sun. 3–6pm
Peterborough	*Tel.* 0733 40515 Tues. 7.30–10pm; Sat. 10am–12 noon
Reading	P.O. Box 9, 17 Catham Street, Reading. *Tel.* 0734 55577 Sun. 7.30–10pm

Rochdale	P.O. Box 9, Rochdale OL16 1OT. *Tel.* 0706 526279 Mon. 7–10pm
Sheffield	P.O. Box 24, Sheffield 1. *Tel.* 0742 755255 Mon. and Fri. 10am–1pm; Thurs. 8–10pm; Sat. 12am–3pm
South Wales	c/o 2 Coburn Street, Cathays, Cardiff. *Tel.* 0222 373181 Mon. and Thurs. 7–10pm; Wed. 11am–12pm
Southampton	P.O. Box 50, Head Post Office, Southampton. *Tel.* 0703 229288 Mon. 7pm–10pm
Strathclyde	P.O. Box 53, Glasgow G2 1YR. *Tel.* 011 221 8448 Mon., Fri., Wed. 7–10pm; Thurs. 11am–1pm
Scunthorpe	P.O. Box 38, Scunthorpe. *Tel.* 0724 853953 Mon. 7–9pm
Swansea	58 Alexander Road, Swansea. *Tel.* 0792 475243 Tues. 7–9pm; Fri. 10am–12 noon
Tyneside	P.O. Box 13, Gosforth, Newcastle-upon-Tyne. *Tel.* (office) 0632 615317 (helpline) 0632 329858 Mon.–Fri. 10am–5pm; Sat. and Sun. 6.30–10pm
Waterford	P.O. Box 57, Waterford, Eire.

Self-help

Women Against Violence Against Women
A Woman's Place,
Hungerford House,
Victoria Embankment,
London WC2
(01 836 6081)

Rape in Marriage Campaign
c/o 374 Grays Inn Road,
London WC1

Scottish Women's Aid
(031 225 8011)

Women Against Rape
London
PO Box 287
London NW6

Bristol
c/o Caroline Barker,
23 Fairlawn Road,
Bristol
(0272 556554)

INCEST: *Recommended reading*
Preventing Child Sexual Assault: a practical guide to talking with children
 by Michele Elliott (Child Assault Prevention Programme) On
 sale from Child Assault Prevention Programme, 26 Bedford
 Square, London WC1B 3HU. Price £1.95 plus 50 pence
 p&p

Self-help
Incest Survivors Group
c/o A Woman's Place,
Hungerford House,
Victoria Embankment,
London WC2
(01 836 6081)

Incest Crisis Line
66 Mariott Close,
Bedfont,
Feltham,
Middlesex
(01 422 5100) (Richard)
(01 890 4732) (Shirley)

CHAPTER TWELVE: GRIEF AND AGEING

BEREAVEMENT *Recommended reading*
Living with Grief by Dr Tony Lake (Sheldon Press)

Self-help
CRUSE
126 Sheen Road,
Richmond,
Surrey PW9 1UR
(01 940 4818)
 (National Organization for the Widowed and their Children)

Society of Compassionate Friends,
5 Lower Clifton Hill,
Clifton,
Bristol
(0272 292778)

Stillbirth and Neonatal Death Society (SANDS)
Argyll House,
29–31 Euston Road,
London NW1 2FD
(01 833 2851)

Foundation for the Study of Infant Deaths (Cot deaths)
The Fifth Floor,
4 Grosvenor Place,
London SW1X 7HD
(01 235 1721/245 9421)

Ageing: Recommended reading
The Art of Ageing by Dr A. Barham Carter (Family Doctor Booklet)
A Good Age by Alex Comfort (Mitchell Beazley)

Epilogue: *Recommended reading*
The Sunday Times Self-Help Directory by Oliver Gillie, Angela Price
   and Sharon Robinson (Granada)

Sex therapy and sex counselling addresses

Almost all the hospitals listed here need a GP referral or a referral from other helping agencies except where otherwise indicated. In addition to these listed addresses most area health authorities (addresses in the area telephone directory) will provide details of psychologists who work in the locality.

Bath	Avon Sex Clinic, Gascoyne House, Upper Borough Walls, Bath *Tel:* Bath (0225) 65593 (Office hours 10am–4pm. Sexual dysfunctions: couples only. Fee in region of £10 per session.)
Birmingham	Department of Psychiatry, University of Birmingham, Queen Elizabeth Hospital, Birmingham B15 2TH *Tel:* 021-472 1301
Bradford	Bradford Royal Infirmary, Psychosexual Clinic, Maternity Unit, Smith Lane, Bradford, West Yorkshire BD9 6RJ *Tel:* Bradford (0274) 42200
Bristol	Department of Psychiatry, Bristol Royal Infirmary, Marlborough Street, Bristol BS2 8HW *Tel:* Bristol (0272) 22041 (Counselling for all sex problems. Waiting list of three months.)
—	Avon Sex Clinic, 21 Richmond Hill, Bristol *Tel:* Bristol (0272) 312316 (Tuesday evenings. Sexual dysfunctions; couples only. Fee in region of £10 per session.)
Doncaster	Doncaster Royal Infirmary, Doncaster *Tel:* Doncaster (0302) 66666
Durham	Department of Clinical Psychology, Winterton Hospital, Sedgefield, Stockton on Tees, Teeside TS21 3EJ (Psychosexual therapy)
Edinburgh	Royal Edinburgh Hospital, Department of Clinical Psychology, Andrew Duncan Clinic, Morningside Terrace, Edinburgh
—	Department of Obstetrics and Gynaecology, Royal Edinburgh Hospital *Tel:* 031-447 2011
Glasgow	Department of Clinical Psychology, Lansdowne Clinic, 3 Whittinghame Gardens, Glasgow G12 0AA *Tel:* 041-334 1734
—	Royal Hospital for Sick Children, University of Glasgow (Clinic for transsexuals)
Hampshire	Nuffield Clinic, Plymouth, Hampshire. Sex therapy: see telephone details in local directory

Ipswich	The Beaumont Trust, 77 Radcliffe Drive, Ipswich, Suffolk *Tel:* Ipswich 0473 59170 (Counselling service for transvestites and transsexuals.)
Kent	Beckenham Hospital, Beckenham, Kent (General sex counselling)
—	Urological Unit, Joyce Green Hospital, Dartford, Kent (Sex problems of a genito-urinary type)
Leicester	Carlton Hayes Hospital, Narborough, Nr. Leicester *Tel:* 053729 2225
London	NHS hospitals dealing with a variety of sex problems
—	St Thomas's Hospital, Lambeth Palace Road, SE1 *Tel:* 01-928 9292
—	Charing Cross Hospital, Fulham Palace Road, W6 *Tel:* 01-748 2050
—	University College Hospital, Gower Street, WC1 *Tel:* 01-387 9300
—	Cassel Hospital, Ham Common, Ham, Richmond, Surrey *Tel:* 01-940 8181
—	Westminster Hospital, Dean Ryle Street, Horseferry Road, SW1 *Tel:* 01-828 9811
—	London Hospital, Whitechapel, E1 *Tel:* 01-247 5454
—	Queen Charlotte's Maternity Hospital, Goldhawk Road, W6 *Tel:* 01-748 4666
—	York Clinic, Guy's Hospital, St Thomas Street, SE1 *Tel:* 01-407 7600
—	St George's Medical School, Psychiatric Research Unit, Aikinson Morley's Hospital, 31 Copse Hill, SW20 *Tel:* 01-946 7711
—	St Olave's Hospital, Lower Road, SE16 *Tel:* 01-237 8275
—	Middlesex Hospital, Mortimer Street, W1 *Tel:* 01-636 8333
—	St Mary's Hospital, Psychosexual Unit Medical School, Praed Street, W1 *Tel:* 01-262 1280
—	Maudsley Hospital, Denmark Hill, SE5 *Tel:* 01-703 6333
—	St Bartholomew's Hospital, West Smithfield, EC1 *Tel:* 01-606 7777
—	King's Family Planning Brook Centre, King's College Hospital, Denmark Hill, SE5 *Tel:* 01-274 6222
Manchester	Withington Hospital, Manchester, M20 8LR *Tel:* (061) 445 8111 (Marital sex therapy, sex counselling and a gender identity service.)

Prescot, Merseyside	Dept Psychological Medicine, Windsor Clinic, (A.T.U.) Rainhill Hospital, Prescot, Merseyside L35 4PQ (General sex problems.)
Middlesbrough	St Luke's Hospital, Middlesbrough, Cleveland TS4 3AF (Sex therapy is available through the psychiatric services. *Any* patient will be accepted.)
Newcastle	Area Psychological Service, Newcastle General Hospital, Westgate Road, Newcastle upon Tyne NE4 6BE *Tel:* Newcastle upon Tyne (0632) 38811 (General help and counselling for people with sex problems; referral by direct enquiry. If long-term treatment is required, the enquirer will need GP's referral. Marital problems are also treated, but there is a waiting list. Department of Psychiatry at Newcastle Hospital specializes in the treatment of trans-sexualism: counselling for transvestites and trans-sexuals is obtainable through the Area Psychological Service.
Northumberland	Department of Psychology, St George's Hospital, Morpeth, Northumberland *Tel:* Morpeth (0670) 2121 (Marital and sexual counselling by the Area Health Authority team of psychologists. In addition to the hospital practice, they also counsel part-time at the surgeries of local GPs.)
Norwich	West Norwich Hospital comes under the Area Psychological Service and provides sex therapy
Rochdale	The Sudden Health Centre, Silk Street, Sudden, Rochdale *Tel:* Rochdale (0706) 58905
Rochford	Rochford General Hospital, Rochford, Essex *Tel:* 0702 544471
Sheffield	University of Sheffield, Department of Psychiatry, Marital and Sexual Difficulties Clinic
—	Whiteley Wood Clinic, Woofindin Road, Sheffield S10 3TL *Tel:* Sheffield (0742) 303901
Southampton	Knowle Hospital, Fareham, Hampshire *Tel:* Fareham (0329) 832271 (Marital sex therapy for couples.)
Surrey	Marital Function Clinic, 3 Ramsey Court, Church Street, Croydon CR0 1RF *Tel:* 01-680 1944 (Offers sex therapy mainly for couples. Fees charged per session. Telephone between 9–1, Mon.–Fri.)
York	Clinic for Psychosexual Disorders, Clifton Hospital, York YO3 6RD *Tel:* York (0904) 24677

Further counsellors specializing in sex therapy and marital counselling may be obtained from:

193

Association of Marital and Sexual Therapists
(Secretary Faye Cooper),
c/o Whiteley Wood Clinic,
Woofinden Road,
Sheffield S10 3TL
(0742 303901)

Bibliography

Bancroft, John and Myerscough, Philip. *Human Sexuality and Its Problems* (Churchill Livingstone)

Barlow, David, *Sexually Transmitted Disease: The Facts* (Oxford)

Fairburn, Christopher G., Dickerson, Mark G., Greenwood, Judy, *Sexual Problems and their Management*

Fallowell, Duncan, *AIDS The Facts, the Fears, the Future* (Sunday Times March 6th. 1985)

Hooper, Anne, *The Body Electric* (Unwin Paperbacks)

Journal of Reproductive Medicine Vol 28 Nos 7 and 8, July–August 1983 Premenstrual Tension: An invitational symposium

Kaplan, Helen Singer, *The New Sex Therapy* (Balliere Tindall)

Kaplan, Helen Singer, *Disorders of Sexual Desire* (Balliere Tindall)

Kellett, John M. *Testosterone; a treatment for low libido in women?* British Journal of Sexual Medicine. April/May 1984

Magos, A. L., Collins, W. P. and Studd, J. W. W. *Management of the Pre-Menstrual Syndrome by Subcutaneous Implants of Oestradiol* Journal of Psychosomatic Obstetrics and Gynaecology, 3 (1984) 93–99

Masters, William H. and Johnson, Virginia E., *Human Sexual Response* (Little, Brown)

Meredith, Sheena, *Recent advances in oral contraception: report of a workshop held at the Royal College of Obstetricians and Gynaecologists* (London (UK) May 6, 1983) British Journal of Sexual Medicine, Sept 1983

Morley, Robert, *Intimate Strangers: a discussion of the psychology of relationships and marriage* (Family Welfare Association 1984)

Morley, Robert, *Separate but Together—the essential Dichotomy of Marriage*, appeared in *Change in Marriage* (National Marriage Guidance Council 1982)

Phillips, Angela and Rakusen, Jill (eds), *Our Bodies Ourselves* (British version) (Penguin)

Riley, Alan, *Androgens and Female Sexuality* (British Journal of Sexual Medicine May 1983)

Yates, Alayne, *Sex Without Shame* (Temple Smith)

Index